W0091541

Indian Systems of Medicine
SKIN DISEASE
(A HERBOMINERAL APPROACH)

Indian Systems of Medicine
SKIN DISEASE
(A HERBOMINERAL APPROACH)

Abdul Hameed

Former Chancellor, AMU, Aligarh; and
Hamdard University, New Delhi - 110062

S.B. Vohora

M.V.Sc., Ph.D., D.Sc.

Reader & Head,
Deptt. of Medical Elementology & Toxicology,
Hamdard University, New Delhi - 110062

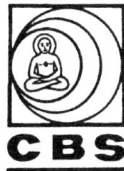

C B S

CBS PUBLISHERS & DISTRIBUTORS

4596/1-A, 11 Darya Ganj, New Delhi - 110 002 (India)
CBS Homepage : http://www.cbspd.com

ISBN : 81-239-0702-8

First Edition : 2001

Copyright © Authors & Publishers

All rights reserved. No part of this publication may be reproduced, stored in a retrieval system, or transmitted in any form or by any means, electronic, mechanical, photocopying, recording, or otherwise, without the prior written permission of the publishers.

Published by S.K. Jain for CBS Publishers & Distributors, 4596/1-A, 11 Darya Ganj, New Delhi - 110 002 (India).

Printed at :
Asia Printograph, Shahdara, Delhi - 110 032

Foreword

It was a pleasure to go through this monograph which describes a new approach to skin care and therapy proposed by Hakeem Abdul Hameed and Dr. S.B. Vohora in the field of skin care. I am reminded of the old saying that *"dust thou art and to dust shalt thou returneth"*. This is particularly relevant in the context of the present work on elementology. It is no secret that the composition of the human body is similar to that of dust. Dr. Vohora has very ably shown the relationship of elements in the physio-pathology of the skin. In this regard, the concept of the new field of elementology is indeed a landmark achievement. The proceedings of the first International Conference on Elements in Health and Disease jointly organized by the World Health Organisation and Institute of History of Medicine and Medical Research (now merged with Jamia Hamdard) at New Delhi in 1983 have opened a new vista for the scientific mind. It is time that more attention is paid to this fascinating study which is full of great promise. The human mind should unravel the secrets of nature in a spirit of unfettered scientific inquiry. An example of such an approach comes to mind in the case of the great Hakeem Late Ajmal Khan of Delhi, who developed the science of facial diagnosis. Unfortunately, this art died with him as there were no successors. The present effort of Hakeem Abdul Hameed and Dr. S.B. Vohora in the field of elementology ranks in this class of refreshingly new approaches to science.

From time immemorial, mankind has been engaged in the quest of external youth and beauty. Sadly, this has been a vain exercise so far, because all matter is subject to decay. None-the-less, this has not deterred the old alchemist from the time of Cleopatra to the present day of multinational companies in providing help to the aging skin. It is noteworthy that these efforts are achieving far greater success than ever before. While the knowledge, talent and equipment is all directed to somehow arrest the aging process, the practical end-objective is only to produce a gracefully aging skin. Towards this objective, we now have several proven methods of treatment starting with creams, ointments, oils etc. to the present day high-tech aspect of lasers, implants of various types, etc. The present monograph has touched on the applications being currently used by women. It is a fact that a large number of cosmetic products being currently sold do contain substances which cause problems to the skin. In the absence of any sophisticated quality control, skin testing procedure, allergic reactions are fairly common. Contact dermatitis through facial cosmetics is an established fact and has led to much misery. In recent years, herbal cosmetics have made their debut with varying claims of success and acceptability. However, this does not mean that herbal cosmetics are devoid of allergy reactions. A new dimension has been added with the use of fruits in cosmetology. Alpha hydroxy acid (AHA) is a good example of fruit ingredient for skin care. The range of products based on fruits have proved very successful and need to be studied further under Indian conditions. It may be noted that these herbal/fruit preparations are being seen through allopathic eyes and are no longer traditional preserves of Unani or other indigenous systems of medicines. It is in such areas of work where there is commonality of concepts and results on the basis of which an integrated programme of research can be conducted by Unani alongwith allopathic doctors. It will go a long way in dispelling some of the misgivings and wrong notions held by allopathic physicians in regard to Unani medicines.

Another important area is in the field of Photochemotherapy applied in the treatment of Leucoderma. The medicine is derived from a plant extract from *Babchi* while the rays used are UVA delivered through sophisticated machines. An integrated approach in this area of work should also be possible for greater efficacy of the treatment.

Dr. Abdul Hameed Rizvi

M.B.B.S. D.D.V. (Vienna) FAMS C SID (London)

Z. Photochemotherapy (Vienna)

Dermatologist-Venereologist and Photochemotherapist

Director

Dr. Rizvi's Skin Clinic & Puva Therapy Research Centre

A-232 Defence Colony, New Delhi 110 024

Preface

According to Dr. P.N. Behl, a famous dermatologist from Delhi about 10 per cent of all hospital cases are skin diseases. The incidence is on the rise with increasing use of chemicals, environmental pollution, occupational exposure and indiscriminate use of cosmetics. Paradoxically the last mentioned preparations are intended for improving the skin complexion and texture but may actually damage it. Skin diseases do not kill but may be associated with severe distress, physical discomfort, irritation, inferiority complex and problems in social acceptability. The treatment necessitates long term therapy. A better understanding of the skin, its composition function and treatment with relatively non-toxic substances such as natural products should, therefore, be advantageous and desirable. Indian systems of medicine (Ayurveda, Siddha and Unani-Tibb) offer a large number of plant, animal and mineral origin drugs and their formulations for use in skin diseases with remarkable claims of efficacy and safety. Some of these claims have been scientifically validated by experimental and clinical studies at Jamia Hamdard and elsewhere. This monograph presents a novel herbo-mineral approach to the understanding and treatment of cutaneous ailments which we believe should be very rewarding if pursued by dedicated investigations with an open mind. If it generates interest in some workers, we will consider our effort to be successful.

The authors gratefully acknowledge help and advice received from many colleagues. Special thanks are due to Dr. H.A. Khan and Prof. M.S.Y. Khan, for elemental analysis data, Dr. M.P. Sharma for help in locating and identifying plant specimens, Mr. A.H. Khan and Mr. Quaiser N. Khan for plant pictures and Mr. Gyan Vikas Mishra for his contribution in Chapter 4. Thanks are due to CCRUM, ICMR and HNF for permission to reproduce certain plant pictures

Abdul Hameed   **S.B. Vohora**

Contents

1

Concept of Impure Blood and Its Purification

1.1 THE QUESTIONS

In Ayurvedic and Unani Tibb skin diseases are attributed to an *impure* status of blood and the treatment is attempted with a class of drugs described as *blood purifiers*. Waheed and Siddiqui[1] listed 46 such drugs: 42 of plant origin and 4 of mineral origin. Many questions come to the minds of people who are not oriented to the traditional concepts (Table 1.1).

Table 1.1: The Questions

- Is there any such thing called *impure* blood?
- If so, how does the blood get impure?
- What precisely is done by so called *blood purifiers* to make it pure?

1.2 AYURVEDIC AND UNANI CONCEPTS

Vaids and *Hakeems* explain it in terms of adverse changes in one or more of body humours. The changes may be brought about by both intrinsic (metabolic) and extrinsic (environmental) factors. Altered properties render the affected humour unfit to perform the specific functions for which it exists in the body or in other words makes the blood impure. Adequate diet, judicious use of herbs, minerals and other natural products, and removal of the cause, are the measures employed to restore purity of blood[2].

1.3 COMMUNICATION GAP BETWEEN TRADITIONAL AND MODERN PHYSICIANS

Unfortunately explanations in terms of changes in humors (bile, black bile, phlegm etc.) and such other theories by traditional physicians are viewed with skepticism and indicted for lack of clarity and scientific evidence. is it really so? Vohora[3,4] felt that the reasons for such attitude lie primarily in the difference of terminology used by the exponents of traditional and modern systems of medicine. He stressed that a *communication gap* exists between the two and there was an urgent need to bridge it. It can be done by more patience and diligent effort on the part of the two systems to try to understand each others philosophy and viewpoint.

1.4 SEARCH FOR EQUATIONS

1.4.1 Impure Blood

To answer the questions listed in Table 1.2 Vohora[3,4] posed some more questions and attempted to answer these.

Table 1.2 What is common between the following conditions?

* Acidosis	* Leukemia
* Allergy	* Lipaemia
* Bacteremia	* Pyaemia
* Cyanosis	* Pyrexia
* Diabetes	* Septicaemia
* Jaundice	* Toxaemia
* Ketonemia	* Uraemia
* Viraemia	

1.4.2 Impurities

It will be seen that in all these conditions, the blood contains: a) such substances which should not be normally present in it or b) an abnormally high concentration of its normal constituents. Some of these are listed in Table 1.3. Obviously the list will be much larger; these are only examples to illustrate the point. The presence of these abnormal substances or of normal substances in abnormal quantities indicates that something has gone wrong with the blood, or in other words, it has become *impure* and the substances listed in Table 1.3 are *impurities*.

Table 1.3 Impurities

* Allergens	* Ketone bodies
* Bacteria	* Sugar
* Fungi	* Bile pigments
* Viruses	* Malignant cells
* Toxins	* Lipids
* Pyrogens	* Methemoglobin
* Pus	* Abnormal metabolic products

1.4.3 Blood purification by Nature

The author[3,4] raised some more questions with the aim of finding suitable equations.

What are the functions of three vital organs: lungs, liver and kidneys? Do they have something to do with blood? The lungs oxygenate the venous blood and return it to the heart via the arteries. The liver has a great role in metabolic processes and detoxifying mechanisms. The kidneys act as special filters to conserve substances wanted by the body, remove the unwanted ones from the blood and eliminate them in urine. They are all guarding against blood impurities. The guards are there within the blood also viz the white blood cells ready to attack the foreign bodies or impurities. The inferences emerging from this discussion are presented in Table 1.4.

Table 1.4 Inferences

* There are *pure* and *impure* states of blood
* The *impure blood* is associated with specific diseases/ailments
* Nature is always alert to purify the blood and restore health.

1.4.4 Blood purification by Man

Are there artificial or man made mechanisms also to purify the blood? Yes, there are. In acute renal failure, for example, the blood is purified by dialysis. The apparatus used is sometimes referred to as the *artificial kidney* because it takes over the functions of the diseased kidneys. The antibiotics and other chemotherapeutic agents purify the blood by destroying the infective agents. The antihistaminic drugs counteract allergens. Various drugs which promote excretory processes (e.g. diuretics, diaphoretics) also aid in purifying the blood. Hypoglycemic and hypochloesterolemic agents bring down excess sugar and cholesterol levels. Anticancer drugs (e.g. *Vinca* alkaloids) destroy malignant cells in leukemias and so on. Thus all attempts (both by Nature and Physician) in diseased states are to restore the *balance of humors, elements and temperaments* or to bring back *homeostasis* from *hyper* or *hypo* states. The difference lies only in the terminology used by traditional and modern physicians and can be equated (Table 1.5).

Table 1.5 The Equation

| Impure Blood | |
Traditional concept	Modern concept
Imbalance/adverse changes in body humors: blood, bile, phlegam, black bile etc.	Disturbance of *homeostasis* leading to *hyper* or *hypo* states, infection, allergy etc.

1.5 BLOOD PURIFYING PLANTS

Vohora[3,4] conducted an exhaustive survey of literature (citing over 100 references) on 36 medicinal plants attributed with blood purifying properties to unearth their relevant pharmacological properties discernible after due scientific scrutiny by experimental and clinical methods. These have been classified into 10 categories and are shown in Table 1.6.

Table 1.6 Pharmacological properties of thirty six blood purifying plants[3]

S.No.	Botanical Name	Unani Name	Relevant Pharmacological Properties
1.	*Acacia catechu,* Willd	*Kattha Safed*	A,B,C,G,H
2.	*Ajuga bracteosa,* Wall	*Nil Kanthi*	D,F,G
3.	*Albizzia lebbeck,* Benth.	*Siras*	A,G,H
4.	*Andrographis paniculata* Nees.	*Kalmegh*	A,B,C,F,H,J
5.	*Bauhinia racemosa,* Lam.	*Kachnal*	G
6.	*Berberis aristata,* DC	*Darhald*	A,B,D,G,H,I,J
7.	*Caesalpinia crista,* Linn.	*Karanjwa*	A,B,C,D,E,I
8.	*Cassia occidentalis,* Linn.	*Kassundi*	A,D
9.	*Celastrus paniculatus, Linn.*	*Malkagni*	A,C,D,I,J
10.	*Cichorium intybus, Linn.*	*Kasni*	I
11.	*Crotalaria juncea,* Linn.	*Senna*	B,G,I
12.	*Curcuma longa, Linn.*	*Haldi*	A,B,E,F,H,I,J
13.	*Dalbergia sissoo,* Roxb.	*Sheesham*	A,B
14.	*Euphorbia hirta,* Linn.	*Dudhi*	A,G,H
15.	*Evolvulus alsinoides,* Linn.	*Sankhavali*	A,B,H
16.	*Fumaria vailantii,* Loisel.	*Shahtara*	A,D,
17.	*Ipomoea turpethum,* R.Br.	*Turbud*	I
18.	*Lactuca scariola,* Linn.	*Kahu*	D
19.	*Lavendula stoechas,* Linn.	*Ustokhuddus*	A,J
20.	*Melia azadirachta,* Linn.	*Neem*	A,B,C,D,E,G,H,I,J
21.	*Mimosa pudica,* Linn.	*Chui Mui*	C
22.	*Nepeta hindustana* (Roth), Haines.	*Badrang Boya*	H,I
23.	*Nerium odorum,* Soland.	*Kaner*	A,G
24.	*Nymphaea alba,* Linn.	*Nilofar*	D
25.	*Ocimum sanctum,* Linn.	*Tulsi*	A,H,J
26.	*Psoralea corylifolia,* Linn.	*Babchi*	A,I,J
27.	*Pterocarpus santalinus,* Linn.	*Sandal surkh*	H
28.	*Rheum emodi,* Wall.	*Revand chini*	I,J
29.	*Rosa damascena,* Mill.	*Gulab*	A,B
30.	*Santalum album,* Linn.	*Sandal safeed*	A,C,J
31.	*Swertia chirata,* Buch.	*Chirayata*	H
32.	*Tephrosia purpurea,* Linn. Pers.	*Sarphooka*	A,D,F
33.	*Terminalia chebula,* Retz.	*Harhar*	A,B,C,D,E,G,H,J
34.	*Tinospora cordifolia* (Willd). Miers.	*Giloe*	A,C,F,G,H,I,J
35.	*Zingiber zerumbet,*Roxb. ex. Smith	*Narkachoor*	A
36.	*Zizyphus vulgaris,* Lam.	*Unnab*	A,H

Abbreviations: A-Antibacterial, B-Antifungal, C-Antiviral, D-Diuretic, E-Anti-allergic/Anti-histaminic, F-Choleretic/hepatotonic, G-Anticancer, H-Hypo-glycaemic/hypocholesterolaemic, I-Anti-inflammatory/antipyretic, J-Adaptogenic and miscellaneous properties.

Frequency distribution of these properties is shown in Table 1.7

Table 1.7 Frequency distribution of pharmacological properties in 36 blood purifying plants[4]

Pharmacological Properties	Number of Plants
Antibacterial	24
Antifungal	11
Antiviral	9
Diuretic	11
Anti-allergic/anti-histaminic	4
Choleretic/hepatotonic	5
Anticancer	11
Hypoglycemic/hypocholesterolemic	15
Anti-inflammatory/antipyretic	12
Adaptogenic and miscellaneous	12

1.6 CONCLUSIONS

It may be concluded that if the Unani term *Musaffi Khoon* be equated with one or more of the 10 categories of pharmacological properties (Table 1.6 and 1.7) and blood impurities with infective agents, allergens, toxins etc. (Table 1.3), the *terminology gap* between traditional and modern systems of medicine will tend to be reduced. A closer understanding between the exponents of various systems is obviously desirable. Let them not fight with each other for superiority but fight the disease.

1.7 REFERENCES

1. Waheed A and Siddiqui HH (1961) *A Survey of Drugs*, ed 2, pp 118-119, New Delhi: Institute of History of Medicine and Medical Research.
2. Ahmad, J (1985) Personal communication
3. Vohora SB (1985) *Hamdard Medicus* **28**(1), 72.
4. Vohora SB (1986) In *Proceedings of the Symposium on Dermatology and Unani System of Medicine* (ed RB Arora), HNF Monograph No. 4, pp. 8-13, New Delhi: Hamdard National Foundation.

2

Role of Elements in the Physiopathology of Skin

2.1 MEDICAL ELEMENTOLOGY

Medical elementology is envisaged as a new discipline in science wherein the number, type, quantity and proportion of elements forms the basis of diagnosis and therapy. It involves a quadrilateral approach which has immense potentialities of development:

i. Elemental composition of the human body in healthy subjects.

ii. Changes in elemental composition in different diseases.

iii. Determination of elements in simple and compound drugs.

iv. Changes in body elements through the use of these drugs during disease states.

The details have been discussed in our earlier publications[1-6].

2.2 ELEMENTAL COMPOSITION OF HUMAN SKIN

Elemental composition of human skin, hair and sweat, reveal the presence of at least 55 elements (Figure 2.1)[7-9]. It is difficult to say how many of these elements are the structural constituents because being the most exposed part of the human body, skin is likely to gather a number of elements from the environment.

2.3 ELEMENTS AFFECTING PHYSIO-PATHOLOGY OF SKIN

A perusal of literature revealed that at least 40 elements affect the physio-pathology of skin (Table 2.1).

Table 2.1 Elements affecting physiopathology of skin

Ag	Al	As	Au	Be	Bi	Br	C
Ca	Cd	Cl	Co	Cr	Cu	Fe	H
Hg	I	K	Mg	N	Na	Ni	O
P	Pb	Pt	Ra	S	Se	Si	Sn
Sr	Te	Th	Ti	Tl	U	Zn	Zr

The effects may be produced by deficiency, excess or medicinal use of these elements or alterations in blood serum or skin concentrations may have potential diagnostic significance.

Skin is 8% of the body weight and uses up about one eighth of body protein. Hence it is affected early in malnutrition. Most malnutrition is a consequence of mixed deficiencies

ESSENTIAL (19)				
C	Ca	Cl	Co	Cu
F	Fe	H	I	K
Mg	Mn	Mo	N	Na
O	P	S	Zn	

POSSIBLY ESSENTIAL (15)				
Al	As	B	Ba	Br
Cr	Ge	Ni	Pb	Rb
Se	Si	Sn	Sr	V

TOTAL (55)

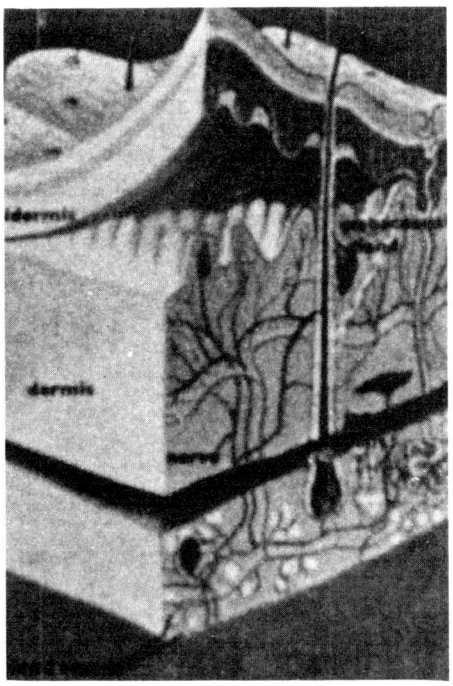

NON-ESSENTIAL (21)					
Ag	Au	Be	Bi	Cd	Cs
Ga	Hg	La	Li	Nb	Po
Ra	Sb	Sc	Sm	Te	Ti
Tl	W	Zr			

Fig. 2.1 Elemental Composition of Human Skin

including those of inorganic elements. Skin diseases of malnutrition have been termed dermatoses of the poor[10]. Contact or exposure to allergens, irritant or caustic elements affects the skin adversely while antiseptic, germicidal and fungicidal properties of some other elements are favourably put to medicinal use. Let us examine the role of individual elements in skin diseases.

2.3.1 Aluminum (Al)

Aluminum compounds have been attributed with antacid, astringent, demulcent and antiperspirant properties[11]. Lotion of Al acetate 1-5% (Burrow's solution) is a popular soak for wet and oozing skin lesions[12]. In hyperhidrosis (excess sweating), the total daily water loss at rest may increase to 12 litres (normal value: about 500 ml). This may even be 3 litres in the first hour; faster than it is possible to drink. Aluminum chloride hexahydrate (20% solution in absolute alcohol) is a specific inhibitor of sweating by acting on openings of the sweat ducts. It is important that the skin be as dry as possible and the patient be tranquil (e.g. at bed time) since dilution of the saturated solution by sweat causes it to become irritant. Supportive therapy to restore water and salt is needed[10].

2.3.2 Arsenic (As)

Inorganic As preparations particularly Fowler's solution have been used for long time for the treatment of psoriasis and other chronic ailments. Occupational exposure may cause chronic As poisoning in workers engaged in manufacture and spray of arsenical pesticides and in Cu smelters. Symptoms manifested in skin include pigmentation, rain drop rash, hyperkeratosis of palms and soles followed by epithelioma of multifocal origin, Black foot disease (dry gangrene) and chronic As poisoning co-occur indicating a cause effect relationship between the two. Data from other than occupational sources support the carcinogenic role of As. Skin lesions (Squamous carcinomas) have been described in some parts of the world with a high As content in drinking water[12-15]. In Unani medicine HARTAL (As-tri-sulphide) is used as a depilatory agent[16].

2.3.3 Beryllium (Be)

Toxic exposures may occur in workers employed in atomic energy, ceramics and fluorescent lamp industries. Direct contact with soluble Be compounds causes contact dermatitis within a few days. Repeated exposures lead to allergic eczematous reaction. If a soluble compound is rubbed into a wound, a chronic indolent ulcer frequently develops which does not heal until the offending material is removed. Accidental implantation of Be phosphor (from a broken fluorescent lamp) has been reported to cause granulomas that must be removed surgically[10,17].

2.3.4 Bismuth (Bi)

In the form of injections (Bisglucol), Bi is useful in syphilis, lichen planus and lupus erythematosus. Prolonged use of Bi can produce lines on the gums and rarely diffuse pigmentation. It is a component of some hair dyes[12].

2.3.5 Bromine (Br)

Bromides produce eruptions resembling ordinary acne or may aggravate existing acne. The lesions appear chiefly on those regions where sebaceous glands are abundant. No commendoes develop; the eruption is frequently associated with mild pruritus. The condition disappears only gradually after the medicament has been discontinued.[12] (Please see also under Sr).

2.3.6 Cadmium (Cd)

Cadmium sulphide (1% suspension) is used in the treatment of seborrhoeic dermatitis. It is not absorbed appreciably from the skin and systemic toxicity has not been reported following its topical use but contact dermatitis may occasionally develop.[18]

2.3.7 Calcium (Ca)

Calcium deficiency may be manifested by itching and white spots on the skin. In systemic treatment of skin disease, Ca-gluconate with or without Vitamin C is used as a non-specific stimulant and desensitising agent[12]. Ointment of unslaked lime (Ca oxide) with animal fat is used in Unani medicine for the treatment of boils. It helps them burst without incision.[16]

2.3.8 Carbon (C)

Carbon di-oxide snow is used for superficial destruction of warts, seborrhoeic warts, cavernous hemangiomas chronic lupus erythematosus, keratoses etc. It is prepared by letting out CO_2 liquid gas from cylinders through a small jet into a Chamois leather bag. As the liquid comes out, snow forms. This is moulded into a pencil. The latter is held between several layers of gauze and applied to the lesions. Carbon arc lamps produce UV rays which are used for the treatment of vitiligo, psoriasis, alopecia aerata and lupus vulgaris.[12]

2.3.9 Chlorine (Cl)

Chlorine is effective at extremely low concentrations (0.0002%) for antiseptic and germicidal actions[17]. Higher concentrations may cause contact urticaria[10]. Workers handling Cl are prone to chlor acne. The lesions occur on the exposed parts of the body and less frequently on the covered areas through contamination of clothes[12].

2.3.10 Chromium (Cr)

McCarthy[19] put forward a hypothesis that because insulin and tolbutamide are therapeutically effective in acne, it rationalizes a recent observation about the value of high chromium yeast in the treatment of acne.

Occupational contact dermatitis can occur from Cr in workers engaged in cement and tanning industries. Chromates may even cause chronic skin ulceration[15]. The rare association of lepromatous leprosy and allergic contact dermatitis due to Cr in cement was confirmed clinically and biologically in a male patient recently[20].

2.3.11 Cobalt (Co)

Sensitivity to Co is commonly found in association with Cr or Ni sensitivity causing metal dermatitis, particularly in hands of women. European standard battery of 24 patch tests for contact dermatitis includes 1% Co-chloride[10].

2.3.12 Copper (Cu)

Copper has a special role in vitiligo or leucoderma (see Chapter 6). Increased serum/plasma levels of ceruloplasmin are a characteristic feature of most infectious diseases[21] including lepromatous leprosy. Copper sulphate possesses antiseptic and fungicidal properties[17,22]. An Unani preparation Kudli Cu gluconate is used for antiseptic, germicidal and fungicidal effects[23].

2.3.13 Gold (Au)

Toxic effects of Au therapy include diffuse slate coloured pigmentation, lichenoid dermatitis, erythema, urticaria and rashes[11,17].

2.3.14 Hydrogen (H)

Hydrogen ion concentration (pH) is an important factor in determining quality of soaps and cosmetics which aught to be pH balanced. Alkaline soap bars may cause skin irritation and precipitation of calcium and fatty acid salts from hard water. Sandal bars are adjusted to pH of normal skin (5 to 6).

2.3.15 Iodine (I)

Tincture and solutions of I are used for the treatment of minor wounds and abbrasions. Idophores are also used for germidical effects. These cause less pain but their efficacy as skin disinfectant is also considerably less than that of 1% I in 70% ethanol[11,17].

2.3.16 Iron (Fe)

Overload of Fe is one of the etiological factors of *Porphyria cutanea tarda* characterised by skin photosensitivity, blistering and scarring pigmentation with hypertrichosis[10].

2.3.17 Lead (Pb)

Lead acetate is used as a hair dye[12] while ointment of Pb carbonate is applied externally for depilatory effect[23] and for the treatment of ulcers and boils[16].

2.3.18 Magnesium (Mg)

A highly significant decrease in serum Mg levels was observed in all clinical types of leprosy including tuberculoid and lepromatous types[24,25].

2.3.19 Mercury (Hg)

Inorganic and organic Hg compounds are used for antiseptic, parasiticidal and fungicidal actions. Recognised supremacy of non-mercurial antiseptics has steadily diminished the use of mercurials. The alkyl and alkoxy Hg compounds are very toxic, cause local irritation and systemic poisoning when absorbed. Hypersensitivity skin reactions may result from the use of mercurial diuretics in some patients. These may vary from mild erythema involving area of contact to severe generalised skin eruptions that may be morbilliform, punctate or urticarial with vesicles and bullae[11]. Mercury vapor lamps are used to produce U.V. light indicated in the treatment of psoriasis, leucoderma, lupus vulgaris and alopecia aerate[12].

2.3.20 Nickel (Ni)

Allergic contact dermatitis may occur in sensitive women from hair pins, cheap jewellery, brassier hooks and other metal fastenings on clothing[12,15]. It may occur in hair dressers from the frequent shampooing affecting their palms. European standard battery of 24 patch tests includes 5% Ni sulphate[10]. Experimental Ni deficiency in chicken, rat and swine causes discoloration, dermatitis and loss of hair. These symptoms could be corrected by Ni supplementation[26,27]. Human deficiency has not been reported.

2.3.21 Nitrogen (N)

Liquid N is a freezing destructive agent, twice as effective as CO_2 snow. It is applied with a cotton tipped applicator on the diseased part while the surrounding skin is protected by a blotting paper. The indications are pale juvenile warts, leukoplakia and capillary hemangioma. On healing minimum atrophy is left behind[12].

2.3.22 Oxygen (O)

Hyperbaric O has been reported to elicit beneficial effect in experimental frost bite[28]. (Please see also under H).

2.3.23 Phosphorus (P)

Yellow P can produce burning on the skin. The affected area should be washed with 1% $CuSO_4$ and dressed as for thermal burns[21].

2.3.24 Platinum (Pt)

Platinum salts cause allergic dermatitis and urticaria in some individuals[10,17].

2.3.25 Potassium (K)

Permanganate of K (1 in 8,000 to 1 in 10,000 solution) is often used for cleaning affected parts in skin diseases. Iodides are used for antiseptic applications. European standard battery of 24 patch tests for dermatitis includes 0.5% K di-chromate solution[10,17].

2.3.26 Radium (Ra)

Beta and gamma rays of Ra are used as surface applicators in selected cases of cavernous hemangioma and epithelioma[12].

2.3.27 Selenium (Se)

In an open trial 29 patients having acne were given 0.2 mg of Se (as Na_2SeO_3) plus 10 mg of tocopherol succinate twice daily for 6-12 weeks. Good results were observed specially in patients with pustular acne and low glutathione peroxidase activity. The enzyme values returned to pre-treatment levels 6-8 weeks after withdrawal of the treatment[29].

Blood glutathione peroxidase (GSH-Px) levels were determined in 61 healthy subjects. Depressed values were observed in patients with psoriasis, eczema, alopic dermatitis, vasculitis, mycosis fungoides, dermatitis herpetiformis, pemphigoid, acne conglobata, polymyositis, rheumatoid arthritis, scleroderma and lupus erythematosus. Fifty six patients with low serum GSH-Px levels were treated with tablets containing 0.2 mg Se (as Na_2SeO_3) and 10 mg tocopherol succinate. Encouraging clinical results were obtained and GSH-Px values increased slowly within 6-8 weeks of treatment[30].

Selenium sulphide (2.5% suspension or shampoo) is used for the treatment of seborrhoeic dermatitis, psorariform seborrhoea, seborrhoea oleosa, acne vulgaris, atopic eczema, tinea versicolor and dandruff. It is not effective in ringworm. It is highly toxic when ingested and so the patients should be advised to wash their hands and clean fingernails to remove traces of drug after each application[12,31]. (Please see also under S).

2.3.28 Silicon (Si)

Seborrhoea is one of the manifestations of experimental Si deficiency in chicken and rat[26]. Human deficiency has not been reported. Silicon barrier creams help in prevention of contact dermatitis[12].

2.3.29 Silver (Ag)

Some Ag compounds (nitrate, allantoinate, sulfadiazine etc) are used for local antiseptic and caustic effects. Chronic Ag poisoning (Argyria) manifests itself (besides other symptoms) by slate blue pigmentation of the elastic fibres of the skin. It starts on face, hands, and finger nails and later becomes generalised. The pigmentation is usually permanent. Nitrate of Ag is also used in hair dyes[11,12,17].

2.3.30 Sodium (Na)

Renal conservation of Na is so efficient that the lowest of salt intakes alone is never enough to induce Na depletion. Deficiency may occur only in cases of abnormal losses from the gut or kidney in disease states. One of the manifestations of Na depletion is reduced skin turgor[32]. Ryan[10] listed Na sulphide and di-oxide salts among the chemicals which cause contact urticaria. Sodium hexa-meta phosphate is an ingredient of a powder mixture used for the treatment of hyperhidrosis[12].

2.3.31 Strontium (Sr)

Strontium bromide (Ekzebrol) has been reported to be useful in eczemoid conditions of filariasis[33].

2.3.32 Sulphur (S)

Sulphur preparations are used in medicine for germicidal, fungicidal and parasiticidal actions. Ointments of S are time honoured remedies for the treatment of acne vulgaris. It is useful for pustules but may not be of much value for commendoes which precede pustulation often by several months[10,17,34]. Therapeutic usefulness of Cd and Se sulphides has been attributed to S; the two metals probably serve as activators. Thus Se may act as an inter-molecular catalyst making the tissue S more active[18]. Unani physicians advocate the use of S bath in scabies and itching[16].

2.3.33 Tellurium (Te)

Industrial exposure to Te fumes and its oxide may cause toxicity which is manifested (besides other symptoms) by suppression of sweating and skin lesions[35]. Tellurium oxide (2.5% suspension/shampoo) is used in the treatment of seborrhoea capitis without local irritation or oiliness of scalp[18].

2.3.34 Thallium (Tl)

Earlier use of Tl acetate as a depilatory agent prior to the treatment of ringworm and epilation in tinea capitis was without medical justification and has been discontinued in favour of fungicidal agents. Dietary levels as low as 0.002% Tl_2O_3 produce alopecia in rats with marked histological changes in skin[12,17].

2.3.35 Thorium (Th)

The main indication of Th is superficial capillary naevus. It emits alpha rays which hardly penetrate 1 mm depth of tissue and has a short half life of about 3 or 4 days. Hence it is difficult to use in practice unless employed near the source of manufacture[12].

2.3.36 Tin (Sn)

Experimental Sn deficiency produced in rats in metal free isolator systems resulted in poor growth, loss of hair, lack of tonicity and a type of seborrhoea. This could not, however, be prevented by Sn supplementation[26]. Tin is used by Ayurvedic physicians for the treatment of skin diseases. This is interesting in view of the fact that there is a tendency for the metal to accumulate in the skin. Large quantities of Sn are retained in the body after oral administration, of which 20-25% is in the skin. It has been observed that workers in Sn mines do not suffer from furuncles and based on this observation stanoxyl was introduced and successfully tried in patients suffering from furunculosis. It may be worthwhile extending these trials in the treatment of such chronic and persisting diseases as eczema, psoriasis etc.[36].

2.3.37 Titanium (Ti)

Titanium tetrachloride is one of the chemicals used as weapons in war. It is a corrosive liquid which decomposes on contact with moist air yielding a dense smoke of Ti-dioxide, Ti-oxychloride and hydrochloric acid. It produces acid burns on skin or eyes[17].

2.3.38 Uranium (U)

Besides radiation effects, uranyl nitrate, U-pentachloride and tetrachloride produce mild to moderate skin irritation[37].

2.3.39 Zinc (Zn)

In malnutrition Zn may be lacking or poorly absorbed. Rough skin is one of the symptoms of Zn deficiency. It is used as an astringent, antiperspirant, styptic and antiseptic agent in the form of lotions, dusting powders or ointments. The compounds used are acetate, chloride, stearate, oleate, permanganate, peroxide and oxide; the last one is most popular. Ointments of ZnO have been used with good results in rash of Kwashiorkor. Severe inflammatory and cystic acne respond to a Zn sulphate citrate complex taken with meals[10,12,17]. Acrodermatitis enterepathica is a well known inherited Zn deficiency disorder exhibiting cerebral, dermal and gastrointestinal symptoms. It responds to oral Zn supplementation both by oral treatment and topical application. Plasma Zn levels were found to be significantly lower (0.25 ± 1 mg/L) in the patients vs the control subjects (0.7 to 1.1 mg/L). After remission following Zn therapy, plasma Zn levels rose to 1.12 ± 0.28 mg/L. Similar changes were observed in Zn concentrations in erythrocytes, hair, skin and urine.

2.3.40 Zirconium (Zr)

Use of Zr salts in cosmetics for anti-perspirant and deodorant actions has been reported. Axillary granuloma may occur from such cosmetics[11,17]. A 4% lotion of Zr dioxide is useful in the treatment of poisoning dermatitis with no systemic toxicity. Clinical trials suggest that preparations of ZrO are useful prophylactically in dermatitis caused by *Rhus* plants as it renders the the active principle of these plants inactive[18].

2.4 CONCLUSIONS: ROLE IN SKIN DISEASES

2.4.1 Deficiency Disorders

A perusal of the foregoing data revealed that deficiencies of Ca, Na, Ni, Si, Sn and Zn result in various skin disorders (Table 2.2).

Table 2.2 Deficiency diseases associated with elemental deficiencies

Element	Disease/Symptoms
Calcium	Itching, White spots
Nickel	Discolouration, Dermatitis, Loss of Hair
Silicon	Seborrhoea
Sodium	Reduced skin turgor
Tin	Loss of hair, Lack of tone, Seborrhoea
Zinc	Rough skin, Acrodermatitis enteropathica

2.4.2 Therapeutic and Diagnostic Use/Potential

At least 26 elements (Ag, Al, As, Bi, C, Ca, Cd, Cl, Cr, Cu, Hg, I, K, N, O, Pb, Ra, S, Se, Si, Sn, Sr, Te, Th, Zn and Zr) find therapeutic applications in a variety of skin ailments (Table 2.3).

Table 2.3 Therapeutic use/potential of elements in skin diseases.

Element	Therapeutic Use/Potential
Aluminum	Antacid Astringent

(Contd.)

	Antiperspirant Oozing skin lesions Hyperhidrosis
Arsenic	Psoriasis Depilatory agent
Bismuth	Syphilis Lichen planus Lupus erythematosus Hair dyes
Cadmium	Seborrhoeic dermatitis
Calcium	Non specific stimulant and desensitising agent Itching White spots Boils

Carbon	CO_2 snow applied on :
	    Warts
	    Seborrhoeic warts
	    Chronic hemangioma
	    Chronic lupus erythematosus
	C arc lamps produce
	UV rays used in :
	    Vitiligo
	    Psoriasis
	    Alopecia aerata
	    Lupus vulgaris

Chromium	High Cr yeast in Acne
Chlorine	Antiseptic Germicidal
Copper	Antiseptic Fungicidal
Iodine	Wounds and abrasions Germicidal
Lead	Hair dye Depilatory agent

Mercury	Antiseptic
	Fungicidal
	Parasiticidal
	Mercury vapour lamps produce UV light used in:
	    Psoriasis
	    Leucoderma
	    Lupus vulgaris
	    Alopecia aerata

(Contd.)

Nitrogen	Liquid N is applied on:
	Pale juvenile warts
	Leukoplakia
	Capillary hemangioma
Oxygen	Hyperbaric O in frost bite
Potassium	Antiseptic
	Germicidal
Radium	Beta and gamma rays in :
	Cavernons hemangioma
	Epithelioma
Selenium	Seborrhoeic dermatitis
	Psorariform seborrhoea
	Seborrhoea oleosa
	Acne vulgaris
	Atopic eczema
	Dandruff
Silicon	Contact dermatitis
Silver	Local antiseptic
	Caustic
	Hair dye
Sulphur	Germicidal
	Fungicidal
	Parasiticidal
	Acne vulgaris
	Scabies
	Itching
Strontium	Eczema associated with filariasis
Tellurium	Sebarrhoea capitis
Thorium	Superficial capillary naevus
Tin	Frunculosis
	Eczema
	Psoriasis
	Chronic skin diseases
Zinc	Acrodermatitis enteropathica
	Astringent
	Antiperspirant
	Antiseptic
	Styptic
	Wound healing
	Rash of Kwashiorkor
	Inflammatory and cystic acne
Zirconium	Antiperspirant
	Deodourant
	Dermatitis due to poisoning and *Rhus* plants

(Contd.)

The diagnostic significance of changes observed in trace element concentration of serum and skin tissue has not been explored. Clear understanding of underlying mechanisms for therapeutic efficacy in many cases is lacking. The role for each and every element present in the skin should be probed carefully. Such knowledge will help in judicious use of elements for a healthy skin.

2.4.3 Adverse Effects

Unfortunately all elements are not begin. Irritant, hypersensitivity, allergic, caustic, pruritic, carcinogenic and other toxic effects may also result from several elements e.g. Ag, As, Au, Be, Bi, Br, Cd, Cl, Cr, Co, Fe, Hg, K, Na, Ni, P, Pt, Te, Ti, Ti, U and Zr. (Table 2.4).

Table 2.4 Adverse effects of elements on skin

Element	Adverse Effects
Arsenic	Skin pigmentation Rain drop rash Hyperkeratosis of palms and soles Epithelioma Black foot disease (dry gangrene) Squamous carcinoma
Beryllium	Contact dermatitis Allergic eczema Granulomas
Bismuth	Diffuse pigmentation
Bromine	Eruptions with pruritus Aggravation of acne
Cadmium	Contact dermatitis
Chlorine	Urticaria Chlor acne
Chromium	Contact dermatitis Chronic skin ulceration
Cobalt	Contact dermatitis
Gold	Slate coloured pigmentation Lichenoid dermatitis Erythema Urticaria Rashes
Iron	*Porphyria cultanea tarda*
Mercury	Hypersensitivity skin reactions Mild erythema Skin eruptions: morbilliform, punctate or urticarial with vesicles and bullae

(Contd.)

Nickel	Allergic contact dermatitis
Phosphorus	Burns
Platinum	Allergic dermatitis Urticaria
Potassium	Dermatitis
Silver	Blue pigmentation of the elastic fibres of skin
Sodium	Urticaria
Tellurium	Suppression of sweating Skin lesions
Thallium	Alpecia Histological changes in skin
Titanium	Corrosive Acid burns
Uranium	Skin irritation Radiation effects
Zirconium	Axillary granuloma

2.5 REFERENCES

1. Vohora SB (1981) *Studies Hist Med* **5**, 61.
2. Vohora SB (1982) *Earth, Elements and Man* Suppl 1, New Delhi: Institute of History of Medicine and Medical Research.
3. Vohora SB (1983) *Medical Elementology* Ed 1, New Delhi: Institute of History of Medicine and Medical Research.
4. Vohora SB (1984) *Curare*, Germany **7**, 155.
5. Vohora SB (1987) *Panchmabhutas* in the light of modern chemistry. Key note address: *Second World Congress on Yoga and Ayurveda*, Varanasi.
6. Vohora SB (1990) In: *New Horizons of Health Aspects of Elements* (an Indo-Polish book), pp 5-14, 143-162, (eds Vohora, SB and Dobrowolski, JW), New Delhi: Jamia Hamdard.
7. Iyenger GV, Kollmer WE and Bowen HJM. (1978) The *Elemental Composition of Human Tissues and Body fluids*, pp 51-54, 100-102, 107-108, New York: Verlag Chemie.
8. Widdowson EM (1965) Chemical analysis of human body. In *Human Body Composition—approaches and applications* (Editor: Brozek, J) pp 31-48, New York: Pergamon Press.
9. Widdowson EM and Dickerson JWT (1964) Chemical composition of the body. In *Mineral Metabolism: An Advanced Treatise* (Eds: Comar CL and Bronner F) Vol 2, Part A, New York: Academic Press.
10. Ryan TJ (1983) Skin diseases. In *Oxford Text Book of Medicine* (Eds: Weatherall DJ, Ledingham JGG and Warrel DA), Vol 2, pp 20 1-30, 98, New York: Oxford University Press.
11. Goodman LS and Gilman A (1975) *The Pharmacological Basis of Therapeutics*, Ed 5, New York: The MacMillan Co.
12. Behl PN (1975) *Practical Dermatology*, Ed 3, Faridabad: Thompson Press (India) Ltd.
13. Doll R and Peto R (1983) Epidermiology of cancer. In *Oxford Text Book of Medicine* (Eds:

Weatherall DJ, Ledingham JGG and Warrelo DA), Vol I, pp 451-478, New York: Oxford University Press.

14. Hopps HC (1971) Geographic pathology and medical implications of environmental geochemistry. In *Environmental Geochemistry in Health and Disease* (Eds: Cannon HL and Hopps HC), pp 1-12, Colorado: The Geological Society of America.

15. Kazantziz G (1983) Occupational exposure to noxious agents In *Oxford Text Book of Medicine* (Eds: Weatherall DJJ, Ledingham JGG and Warrel DA), Vol 1 pp 6-996.115, New York: Oxford University Press.

16. Ummul Fazal and Razzack MA (1976) *A Hand Book of Common Remedies in Unani System of Medicine*, pp 127-132, New Delhi: Central Council of Research in Indian Medicine and Homeopathy.

17. Dipalma JR (1965) *Drill's Pharmacology in Medicine* Ed 3, New York: Mcgraw Hill BGook Co.

18. Krantz JC and Carr CJ (1965) *The Pharmacologic Principles of Medical Practice*, Ed 6, p 197 Calcutta: Scientific Book Agency.

19. McCarthy M (1984) *Medical Hypotheses* **14(3)**, 307.

20. Jerez J, Quintanilla E. Martin-Gil D *et al* (1980) *Dermatologica* **160(1)**, 30.

21. Beise WR (1972) *Amer J Clin Nutr* **25**, 1254.

22. Goulding R (1983) Poisoning from chemicals, In *Oxford Text Book of Medicine* (Eds: Weatherall DJ Ledingham JGG and Warrel DA). Vol 1 p. 6, 15, New York: Oxford University Press.

23. Wahid A and Siddiqui HH (1961) *Survey of Drugs* Ed 2, p 16 New Delhi: Institute of History of Medicine and Medical Research.

24. Nigam P, Dayal SG, Srivastava P *et al* (1979) *Asian J Infect Dis*, **32**, 81

25. Sinha S.N., Gupta SC and Bishi D (1978) *Lepr India* **50 (1)**, 54.

26. Mertz (1974) *Proc Nutr Soc*, **33 (3)**, 307.

27. Nielsen FR (1976) Newer trace elements and possible applications in man In *Trace Elements in Human Health and Disease* (Eds, Prasad AS and Oberleas D), Vol 2 pp 379-400, New York: Academic Press.

28. Bal Krishan, Hedge KS and Mathew L (1978) *Def Sci J* **28 (2)**, 87.

29. Michaeleson G and Edqvist LE (1978) *Arch Derm Venerol* **64 (1)**, 19.

30. Juhlin L, Edqvist LE, Ekman LG *et al* (1982) *Acta Derm Venerol* **62 (3)**, 211.

31. Sanchez JL and Torrers VM (1984) *J Amer Acad Dermatol* **11 (2ptI)**, 235.

32. Ledingham JGG 91983) Water and electrolyte disturbances. In *Oxford Text Book of Medicine* (Eds: Weathrall DJ, Ledingham JGG and Warrel DJ), Vol 2, p. 18.25. New York: Oxford University Press.

33. Sahu, KC and Jena, DC (1967) *Indian Practnr* **20(1)**, 121.

34. Srivastava OP (1969) *J Sci Industr Res* **18 C**, 25.

35. Fishbein L (1977) Toxicology of Selenium and Tellurium. In *Toxicology of Trace Elements* (Eds: Goyer RA and Mehlman MA) Vol 2, pp 191-240, New York: John Wiley and Sons.

36. Chopra RN, Chopra IC, Handa KL et al (1958). *Chopra's Indigenous Drugs of India* p. 445, Calcutta: U.N. Dhur and Sons Pvt. Ltd.

37. Yuile CL (1973) Animal experiments. In *Handbook of Experimental Pharmacology: XXXVI Uranium, Plutonium Transplutonic Elements* (Eds: Hodge HC, Standard JN and Hurrh JB), p. 171, Berlin: Springer Verlag.

38. Anttila P, Salmela S, Simell O et al (1984) In *Proceedings of the First International Conference on Elements in Health and Disease* (Eds Vohora SB and MSY Khan), p. 257, New Delhi: WHO and Institute of History of Medicine and Medical Research.

39. Ohlsson A (1980) *Acta Pediatr Scand* **70(2)**, 269.

40. Parra CA and Smalik AV (1981) *Dermatogica* **163(5)**, 413..

3

Cosmetics from Nature

3.1 BEAUTY IS NOT SKIN DEEP

The urge to look attractive is not new but people are becoming more beauty conscious these days. What makes a person look attractive? Pimples, black heads, blemishes, pock marks, baldness, greying of hairs, wrinkles, ravages of age etc are frequent sources of anxiety and psychological distress. Keeping the genetic makeup, racial differences and pleasing manners aside, glowing health and a vibrant youthful body are obviously the most important factors. A healthy person in the prime of youth should need no external aids to look presentable except, of course, the observance of general rules of self care and hygiene. A famous dermatologist[1] stated: "Skin disease may be indicative of another underlying malaise. Skin is an organ, the largest one in fact, and should be handled with respect. It acts as a mirror, reflecting disease of other organs e.g. the pallor of anaemia, the yellow tinge of jaundice, the blue hue of heart disease, darkening due to chronic infections and adrenal diseases, dysmorphophobia and dermatitis artefacto due to psychological factors etc". In these cases the cause has to be looked into to restore normal health.

3.2 EXTERNAL AIDS: ARE THESE SAFE?

3.2.1 Adverse Effects of Strong Cosmetics

External aids, are, unfortunately, a necessity for others. How do we choose these aids? What kind of soaps, shampoos and oils should we use? What is the impact of an indiscriminate use of too much cosmetics and beauty aids on ones health and personality? Let us look into these questions and problems.

According to Shahnaz Hussain, a well known expert on beauty and skin care, strong soaps and shampoos remove the natural oil from skin and hair, aggravate dryness and cause loss of lustre[2]. A simple mildly alkaline soap should be chosen. Strong medicated soaps should be avoided as these are least useful as medication, can be great sensitizers and may be toxic in certain situations. The use of soap is absolutely forbidden in acute inflammatory conditions, particularly in those that are eczematous[3]. There are controversial reports about the dangers of hexachlorophene (a strong germicidal and deodourizer) in soaps, shampoos, talcum powders and other cosmetics and toiletries. It has even been indicted for episodes of infant mortality in France. The use of caustic materials (sodium and potassium hydroxide) in soaps may cause irritant effects, particularly in delicate skin of children, corners of eyes, mucus membranes, eroded and injured skin, burns and may cause accidental poisoning[4-6]. Shampoos, perfumed oils, depilatory agents and dyes may cause allergic reactions. That is why their information folders advise prior patch test (at the back of the ear or neck) for sensitivity. Vegetable dyes are usually the safest. In Europe and America, cosmetics are responsible for a great deal of contact eczema. The incidence in Asiatic countries is fortunately low but there are reports indicating a recent spurt in cosmetic-induced dermatitis cases in India, particularly in urban areas[3].

3.2.2 The Vicious Cycle

Thick coats of make up with a parapehernalia of lotions, creams, powders, face packs, lipstick, rouge, mascara, eye-shadows, vermilon, perfumes etc. do not make a person attractive or desirable. On the contrary, their effect is more often repulsive. These coatings, besides looking aweful, have adverse effects. They cause blocking of numerous pores of the skin and interfere in its normal secretory and excretory functions. This interference with the physiological mechanisms takes away the normal opportunity from the skin to maintain its health. As a result it looses its smoothness and lustre necessitating more cosmetics to put up a false facade. The vicious cycle continues. How do we escape from it?

3.3 COSMETICS FROM NATURE

3.3.1 The Golden Rule

The golden rule is to avoid artificial aids to look beautiful. Health has no substitute and it can be attained only through balanced nourishing diet, proper hygiene and active habits. But this is easier said than followed in present day circumstances. Minimum use of cosmetics and toiletries with maximum safety is the next alternative. Cosmetics from Nature (e.g. plant and food-based substances) provide the answer to the problem. Obviously the body is more accustomed to these than it can ever be to synthetic chemicals. An association of centuries and generations is bound to make the system more attuned to natural products.

3.3.2 Ancient Heritage

Let us look back at our ancient heritage, What were the beauty aids of royal maidens, princesses, queens, lovely courtesans and dance girls? Many of these were simple items we are all familiar with. Some examples are almonds, seasame, bengal gram flour, maize flour, henna leaves, sandal wood, turmeric, rose flowers, citrus fruit juices and peels, milk, yoghurt, honey etc. The preparations included *ubtans* applied to the body before taking fragrant baths. These were meant to clear the skin of blemishes and improve its texture and complexion. Massage oils were used to tone up the system and make the skin wrinkle-free and youthful. Herbal hair washes were taken to promote growth of soft, black and lusterous hair. Some of these formulae are still used in Indian households as the knowledge of recipes has been passing from mothers to daughters for generations. Readymade herbal cosmetics and toilet goods have also come into being for convenience. Fashionable beauty parlours are making extensive use of formulae and beauty aids known to ancient people.

3.3.3 Herbal Skin Care Products

A recent seminar organized by Central Institute of Medicinal and Aromatic Plants, Lucknow[7] revealed that more than 113 pharmacies are manufacturing at least 439 skin care related products in India (Table 3.1).

Table 3.1 Herbal skin care products manufactured in India.[7]

Category/Use	Number
Enhancement of beauty (face packs, cleansing creams)	4
Stimulating wound healing (ointments, lotions, dusting powders)	13
Care of gums and teeth (tooth powders, tooth pastes, applicants for tooth ache, bleeding gums, mouth washes).	30
Antiaging products (Capsules, tablets, liquids, creams for internal and external use)	41
Pain relieving agents (ointments, balms, creams, rubs, tablets, liquids, for external and internal use)	66
Hair-care products (oils, liquids, creams, dyes, shampoos, antidandruff agents, hair growth promoters)	88
Skin care products (creams, lotions, pastes, powders, ointments, capsules, pills for external and internal use for healthy and diseased skin)	177
Total	439

A majority of these products are intended for use in healthy state and so fall under the category of cosmetics. The lists of manufacturers and products are obviously not exhaustive; the actual number is estimated to be much higher. It indicates the disillusionment of users with synthetic cosmetics and a growing trend of *coming back to nature* for skin and hair care.

3.4 SHORT SCIENTIFIC NOTES ON SOME SIMPLE INGREDIENTS USED IN HERBAL COSMETICS

A perusal of the ingredients of these products shows that these contain besides medicinal herbs and some mineral constituents, very simple and familiar item commonly encountered in kitchen and domestic use.

Short scientific notes on some of the ingredients used are given below:

3.4.1 Almonds (*Prunus amygadalis*)

Oil of almonds is reported to possess demulcent, emollient, stimulant and nervine tonic properties. Its actions are similar to that of olive oil and is used by pharmaceutical and cosmetic industry in nourishing cold creams for the skin as also in superfatted soaps. Kernels are very nutritious and calorie-rich. Chemical composition of the kernels is given below[8].

Moisture	5.2%
Protein	20.8%
Fat (Ether extract)	58.9%
Fibre	1.7%
Mineral matter	2.9%
(Ca, P, Fe, Na, K, Mg, Mn, I, Zn, As, etc.)	
Thiamine	0.24 mg/100 g
Nicotinic acid	2.5 mg/100g
Riboflavin	0.15mg/100 g
Vitamin A	Absent
Vitamin C	Absent

Protein concentrate of almonds contains *amandinas* as the chief protein. It is a globulin (with 19% N content) containing several essential amino acids (e.g. arginine, histidine, lysine, phenyl alanine, leucine, valine, tryptophan, methionine, cystine etc.) that may be needed for nourishment of the body. It is important to note that gamma globulin fraction of the plasma contains antibodies and is credited with resistance mechanisms against infections. Poultice of kernels is reported to be useful in irritable sores and skin eruptions.[8-10]

A crystalline compound isolated from almond shells (identity not established) has been shown to elicit pronounced anti-bacterial action against *Pseudomonas pyocyanea*. Its minimum effective concentration is 1:500. Pure compound exerted the effect within 5 minutes but bactericidal action was seen only after 15 minutes if a dilution of 1:20 was used[11].

3.4.2 Seasame (*Sesamum indicum*)

The oil possesses emollient properties and is claimed to be useful in piles and as a poultice in ulcers. The seasame protein concentrate forms a good protein for any *ubtan* or massage oil for nourishing and stimulating the skin. A complex cyclic ether (seasamin) isolated from the seeds is reported to elicit anti-tubercular activity. The effect was observed in 1:10 million dilution and it lasted for 3 weeks[10,12].

3.4.3 Turmeric (*Curcuma longa*)

Dried pulverised rhizomes are used. It is one of the most extensively investigated plant based drug and is reported to possess antibacterial, antifungal, antiallergic/anti-histaminic, hypocholesterolaemic and antioxidant actions due to the phenolic character of curcumin. Of its various actions, its anti-inflammatory effects are most potent. The drug is used for various inflammatory conditions and also for promoting healing process of fractures. Beneficial effects of turmeric have been reported in histamine-induced gastric ulcers in experimental animals.[9,13-17]

3.4.4 Bengal Gram Flour (*Cicer arietinum*)

Dried pulverized grains are used. It is attributed with nourishing and astringent properties. Whole Bengal gram contains (per 100 g.):

Proteins	17.1 g
Fat	5.3 g
Carbohydrates	60.9 g

Calories	360
Thiamine	300 mg
Riboflavin	510 mg
Nicotinic acid	2.1 mg
Calcium	202 mg
Iron	10.2 mg
Magnesium	168 mg
Phosphorus	312 mg
Sodium	37 mg
Potassium	808 mg
Arsenic	9 μg

Presence of carotenoids and oil soluble Vitamins A, D and E has been reported[9,10,18,19]

3.4.5 Maize Flour *(Zea mays)*

Dried pulverized grains are used. It is attributed with resolvent and astringent properties. Presence of anti-bacterial substances has also been reported in maize seeds. Dried maize contains (per 100 g):

Proteins	11.1 g
Fats	3.6 g
Carbohydrates	66.2
Calories	342
Thiamine	420 μg
Riboflavin	10 μg
Nicotinic acid	1.4 mg
Calcium	10 mg
Iron	2 mg.
Magnesium	144 mg
Phosphorus	348 mg
Sodium	16 mg
Arsenic	30 μg

Maize flour is reported to facilitate iron absorption[9,10,20]

3.4.6 Sandal Dust *(Santalum album)*

Dried pulverised wood is used or wood as such is ground with water to yield a paste. The paste is applied to forehead and temples for soothing effect. It is claimed to cure headache, fevers, itching and local inflammation. Oil from heart wood is said to be useful in gonorrhoeal urethritis, cystitis and skin diseases. Scientific evidence of its antibacterial and antiinflammatory effects is available in some reports[10,22,23]. Sandalwood improves the normal functions of skin by influencing it at the cellular level. Its paste and scent are soothing to nerves and induce relaxation. According to Shahnaz Husain[24], a relaxed mind is a prerequisite for beauty and so it makes the cosmetic treatment more effective in acne and pimples. It is ideal for oily skin and seborrhoeic conditions. Red sandalwood protects the skin from sun damage and is, therefore, incorporated in sun screens and sun protective creams for use in prickly heat and rashes. Sandal dust blends well with other oils and extracts and can easily be added to various cosmetic preparations.

3.4.7 Citrus fruit Peels (e.g. *Citrus reticulata*)

Oil from peels contain d-limonene terpene, carene, linalool etc. The fruits are a rich source of Vitamin C which has a significant role in increasing body resistance to diseases. Pectins, aurantin (a fully methylated flavonol), glycosides, flavonoids and anti-hyaluronidase enzyme are also reported present. Aglycone and flavonoidal principles present in citrus fruits peels are reported to possess antimicrobial properties. It is believed to exert a bleaching action which helps in clearing blemishes and improving complexion[10,17,25-27].

3.4.8 Rose Petals (*Rosa damascena*)

Besides being pleasantly fragrant, rose petals are reported to possess antibacterial and antifungal properties[28,29]. Incorporation of the essence in lotions, creams and soaps may, therefore, have a beneficial effect in skin infections.

3.4.9 Honey (*Mel*)

Honey because of its highly hygroscopic nature, elicits good antimicrobial activity. It is highly nutritious and contains:

Moisture	17%	
Sugars	64%	(Levulose 39%, Dextrose 34%, Sucrose 1%)
Dextrin	0.5%	
Proteins	2%	
Wax	1%	
Mineral salts	1%	(Al, Ca, Cl, Cu, Fe, I, K, Mn, Na, PO_4, S, Si etc.)

Resins, gums, pigments, pollen grains, enzymes and vitamins (Thiamine, Ascorbic acid, Riboflavin, Pentothinic acid, Pyridoxine, Niacin, Vitamin K etc.) are also present. The use of honey has been mentioned in face creams and lotions to remove wrinkles and blemishes, in the treatment of burns (leaving no scar), fruncles, boils and for soothing effect in irritant inflammatory conditions. An International Symposium on Apitherapy was organized in Poland wherein several papers on therapeutic effects of honey and other bee products were presented[8,30,31]. Studies carried out at Jamia Hamdard on Polish propalis bee products, revealed good antibacterial (particularly against gram negative organisms), antifungal (against fungi responsible for superficial and dermatomycoses) and anti-inflammatory (against acute and chronic models of inflammation) effects[32].

3.4.10 Milk and Yoghurt (*Lactus*)

These are attributed with nourishing, cleansing and soothing effects. Traditional use of milk and yoghurt for washing hair and face before bath is not without scientific basis. These products help in restoring the natural oil of skin and hair making them soft, smooth and lusterous[33].

Nature is an inexhaustible mine from which innumerable products can be unearthed for use as cosmetics. A few examples are cited above to illustrate the point.

3.5 REFERENCES

1. Panja, R.K. (1985): Miscellany, *Times of India* Sept. 1.
2. Hussain S (1985): *Times of India*, Sunday Review, 25 August, p. 5.
3. Behl PN (1975): *Practice of Dermatology*, Ed. 3, New Delhi: Thomson Press (India) Ltd..
4. Anonymous (1955): *The Dispensatory of the United States of America*, Ed. 25, pp. 1275-76, Toronto: JP Lippincott Co.
5. Anonymous (1979): *The British Pharmaceutical Codex*, Ed. 11, p. 828, London: Pharmaceutical Press.
6. Martindale (1982): *Extra Pharmacopoeia*, Ed. 28, p. 45, London: The Pharmaceutical Press.
7. *National Seminar on the Use of Traditional Medicinal Plants in Skin Care* Central Institute of Medicinal and Aromatic Plants, Lucknow, November 25-26, 1994.
8. Anonymous (1948-1976): *The Wealth of India*, vols. I-XI, New Delhi· Council of Scientific and Industrial Research.
9. Antia FP (1973): *Clinical Dietetics and Nutrition*, Delhi: Oxford Press.
10. Chopra RN Nayar SL and Chopra, IC (1956): *Glossary of Indian Medicinal Plants,* New Delhi: Council of Scientific and Industrial Research.
11. Gupta U, Bhatia VN, Venugopal P et al (1971): *Indian J. Med. Res.*, **59**, 1002.
12. Ramaswamy, AS and Sirsi M (1957): *Die Naturwise enhcaften*, **44**, 1.
13. Basu AP (1971): *Indian J. Pharm.*, **33(6)**, 127.
14. Bhatia A Singh GB and Khanna NM (1964): *Indian J. Exp. Biol.*, **2**, 158.
15. Dineschandra and Gupta SS (1972): *Indian J. Med. Res.*, **60(1)**, 138.
16. Pachauri SP and Mukherjee SK (1970): *J. Res. Indian Med.*, **5(1)**, 27.
17. Vohora SB (1985): *Hamdard Medicus* **28(1)**, 72.
18. Madhwan M Chandra K and Reddy DJ (1971): *Indian J. Med. Sci.*, **25**, 771.
19. Mathur KS, Khan MA and Sharma R (1968): *Brit. Med. J.*, **1**, 30.
20. Moore CV and Dubach R (1956): *J. Amer. Med. Asso.*, **162**, 197.
21. Shende ST, Balasundaram VR and Sen A (1968): *Indian J. Microbiol.*, **3(2)**, 143.
22. Jain SK (1975): *Medicinal Plants*, Ed. 2, p. 125, New Delhi: National Book Trust.
23. Srimathi RA and Sreenivasaya M (1963): *Curr. Sci.*, **32(1)**, 11.
24. Husain S (1995): Health column. *Hindustan Times*, June 28, p. 16.
25. Ghose BP (1958): *Indian J. Med. Sci.*, **12**, 991.
26. Ramaswamy AS, Jayraman S, Sirsi M et al (1972): *Indian J. Ex. Biol.*, **10**, 72.
27. Sarin JPS, Mitra RK, and Ray GK (1960): *Indian J. Pharm.*, **22(9)**, 234.
28. Dixit SN and Tripathi SC (1975): *Indian Phytopath.*, **28(1)**, 141.
29. Okazak K and Oshima S (1953): *J. Pharmaceut. Soc. Japan*, **73**, 344.
30. *International Symposium on Apitherapy* (1985): Krakow (Poland), May 23-26.
31. Norris, P (1969): *About Honey,* London: Thornson Publications.
32. Dobrowolski JW, Vohora SB, Sharma K et al (1991): *J Ethnpharmacology*, **55**, 77.
33. Vohora SB and Khan MSY (1978): *Animal Origin Drugs Used in Unani Medicine*; Ed. 1, pp. 32-34, 102, New Delhi: Institute of History of Medicine and Medical Research and Vikas Publishing House.

4

Herbal Dermatology : Plants and Formulations Used and Their Rationale*

4.1 RATIONAL BASIS OF THE USE OF MEDICINAL PLANTS IN SKIN DISEASES

A large number of medicinal plants are claimed to be useful in skin diseases in all traditional systems of medicine and folklore. While these plant remedies (both single plants and multi-herbal formulations) are being used orally and by local application since ancient times, the mechanisms whereby such effects are elicited have not been looked into. These effects may be brought about by their inherent antibacterial (A), antifungal (B), antiviral (C), antiinflammatory (D), wound healing (E), antiallergic/antihistaminic (F) and anticancer (G) properties or through the content of vitamins A,C and E in these plants (H). The effects may also be attributed to their blood purifying (I) and adaptogenic (J) properties. A survey of literature revealed that such properties were reported in at least 455 medicinal plants with claimed utility in skin diseases (Table 4.1). The frequency distribution of relevant activities reported in these plants is presented in Table 4.2 and 4.3. The following observations emerge from a perusal of these tables:

i.   Majority of the plants exhibited only one (50%) or two (25%) types of pharmacological activities considered relevant to skin diseases. None of the plants revealed more than 7 type of activities listed.

ii. Antimicrobial (anti-bacterial, anti-fungal, anti-viral) properties topped the list (about 60%), followed by vitamin containing plants (25%), antiinflammatory, anticancer, and adaptogenic (approximately 20% plants in each category) properties. Plants with other

*This chapter was prepared jointly with Mr Gyan Vikash Mishra, Ph.D Scholar and UGC Fellow working in the Department of Medical Elementology and Toxicology, Jamia Hamdard.

type of reported pharmacological actions ranged between 1-14% of the 463 plants surveyed. While no claim is being made of an exhaustive survey of literature on the subject. The present review with 226 references gives a fair representation of the pharmacological properties of plants reputed to be of therapeutic value in traditional dermatology.

iii. Scientific confirmation of such wide range of relevant pharmacological properties in these plants indicates that their traditional use in skin diseases has some rational basis.

iv. The reports cited in the review were not aimed specifically to search plant remedies with dermatological value. Planned experimental and clinical studies on these aspects are not available. These are obviously warranted and might be very rewarding.

Table 4.1 Medicinal Plants used in skin diseases with relevant pharmacological properties

Abbreviations:

A-Antibacterial;	B-Antifungal;	C-Antiviral;
D-Antiinflammatory;	E-Wound healing;	F-Antiallergic/antihistaminic;
G-Anticancer;	H-Containing vitamins A,C and E;	I-Blood purifying;
J-Adaptogenic/antiageing properties.		

S. No.	Plant	Activities Reported	References
1.	*Abies alba* Mill	E	1
2.	*Abrus precatorius* Linn	B, G	2-4
3.	*Acacia sp.* Willd	A, B, C, D, G, I	2, 7-15, 21, 174, 175, 180-181
4.	*Acanthospermum hispidum* DC	A	16
5.	*Achillea millefolium* Linn	J	7
6.	*Achyranthes aspera* Linn	A	3
7.	*Aconitum heterophyllum* Wall	J	7
8.	*Acorus calamus* Linn	J	7
9.	*Adhatoda vesica* Nees	C, J	2,.7
10.	*Adhatada zeylanica* Nees	D	17
11.	*Aegle marmelos* Correa	C	2, 7, 9
12.	*Aesculus hippocastanus* Linn	C	7
13.	*Ajuga bracteosa* Wall	G, I	2, 8, 9, 18
14.	*Albizzia lebbeck* Benth	A, D, F, G, I	2, 3, 8, 9, 19, 20
15.	*Albizzia procera* Benth	C, G	6, 21

(Contd.)

S. No.	Plant	Activities Reported	References
16.	*Alectra parasitica* A Rich	A	9, 22, 23
17.	*Alianthus excels* Roxb	A	24
18.	*Allium cepa* Linn	G, H	14, 25
19.	*Allium sativum* Linn	A, C, D, E, H, I	1-3, 8, 14, 25, 27, 28, 30
20.	*Alnus nitida* Engl	C	31
21.	*Aloe* Sp.	E, G, I	2, 3, 7, 8, 177
22.	*Alpinia* Sp.	A, B, C, D, G	5, 7, 14, 32
23.	*Alstonia scholaris* Roxb	G	3
24.	*Alringia excelsa* Noronha	C	27
25.	*Amelia asiatica*	J	7
26.	*Amomum subulatum* Roxb	C, J	7
27.	*Amura rohitaka* Wright & Arn	A, C, G	3
28.	*Anacardium occidentale* Linn	G	3
29.	*Anacyclus pyrethrum* DC	A, J	7
30.	*Anagallis arvensis* Linn	A	3
31.	*Anamirta coculus* Wright & Arn	G.	2, 15, 21, 33
32.	*Andrographis paniculata* Nees	A, B, C, J	2, 10, 34-37
33.	*Angelica polyclada* French	H	7
34.	*Annona squamosa* Linn	A, G	3, 5, 7, 21
35.	*Antidesma menasu* Miq	D	28
36.	*Aphnamixis polystachys* Pasker	D, G	3, 7, 9, 17
37.	*Aquilaria agallocha* Roxb	J	7
38.	*Arachis hypogea* Linn	H	7
39.	*Arctium lappa* Linn	H	7
40.	*Areca catechu* Linn	A, B	3, 40
41.	*Argimone mexicana* Linn	A, C	3, 9, 42
42.	*Argemone ochraleuca* Sweet	G	41
43.	*Argyreia involucrata* Clarke	G	15, 21
44.	*Argyreia speciosa* Sweet	D, J	7, 28
45.	*Aristolochia indica* Blanco	E	2, 8
46.	*Arnebia hispidissma* Vanot	D	28
47.	*Arnebia nobilis* Rach	A, B, G	3, 14, 21, 38
48.	*Arnica sp*	E	7
49.	*Artemisia absinthium* Linn	A, C, E	1, 5, 8, 174
50.	*Artemisia parviflora* Buch	E	31
51.	*Artemisia scoparia* Weldst et Kit	A	5
52.	*Asparagus officinalis* Linn	H	25
53.	*Asparagus racemosus* Willd	G, J	3, 7, 9

(Contd.)

S. No.	Plant	'Activities Reported	Reference
54.	*Astercantha longifolia* Nees	A, B, H, J	3, 7, 43
55.	*Atlantia racemosa* Corr	C	3
56.	*Avena sativa* Linn	H, J	7
57.	*Azadirachta indica* Juss	A, B, C, D, E, F, G, I, J	3, 7, 8, 14, 21, 28, 30, 38, 42, 44, 45, 70, 71, 117-128, 178, 224
58.	*Bacopa monnieri* Linn	G, H, J	3, 7, 21, 38
59.	*Bambusa arundinacea* Druce	A	2, 7
60.	*Bauhinia racemosa* Lam	G, I	2, 3, 8, 9
61.	*Berberis aristata* DC	A, B, D, E, G, H, I, J	2, 3, 7, 8, 9, 28, 29, 46-48, 174
62.	*Berberis asiatica* Grift	G	9
63.	*Berberis macrozepata* Hook f	b	17
64.	*Berginia ciliata* Blatter	G	3
65.	*Berginia ligulata* Engl	D	28
66.	*Betula alba* Linn	A, I	7
67.	*Bixa orellano* Linn	H	7
68.	*Blighia sepida* Kon	D	28
69.	*Blumea* Sp.	A	14, 52
70.	*Boerhaavia diffusa* Linn	D, H, J	2, 3, 7, 28
71.	*Borassus flabellifer* Linn	H, I	2, 8, 25
72.	*Boswelia serrata* Roxb	D, G	3, 28
73.	*Brassica* Sp.	H	7, 25
74.	*Bridelia retusa* Spreng	C, G	6, 21
75.	*Brunello vulgaris* Linn	H	7
76.	*Butea monosperma* Tausert	D	28
77.	*Caccinia glauca* Savi	D	28
78.	*Caesalpinia bonducella* Flem	A, C	3, 5, 9, 28, 53
79.	*Caesalpinia crista* Linn	A, B, C, D, F	5, 7, 17, 28, 54-58
80.	*Caesalpinia sepiaria* Roxb	C	38
81.	*Calendula officinalis* Linn	E, H	7
82.	*Calophyllum inophyllum* Linn	A, D	28, 59
83.	*Calotropis gigantea* Roxb	G	3, 9, 21
84.	*Calotropis procera* Ait f	A,G,J	3,7,21,60
85.	*Cannabis sativa* Linn	J	7
86.	*Capparis decidua* Edg	A, B, C, J	3, 7, 61, 62, 65
87.	*Capparis grandis* Linn f	G	33
88.	*Capsicum annum* Linn	H	25
89.	*Capsicum minimum* Roxb.	E	7
90.	*Cardiospermum helicacabum* Linn	A	66
91.	*Carica papaya* Linn	C, H	2, 7, 25
92.	*Carissa carandus* Linn	A	3
93.	*Carum carvi* Linn	H, J	7
94.	*Caryophyllus aromaticus* Linn	H, J	7
95.	*Cassia absus* Linn	A, D	3, 28, 182
96.	*Cassia alata* Linn	B, D, E	2, 7, 14, 15, 21
97.	*Cassia angustifolia* Vahl	B, D, I	2, 3, 8, 28, 68, 100, 174, 176
98.	*Cassia auriculata* Linn	C	3, 9, 14

(Contd.)

S. No.	Plant	Activities Reported	Reference
99.	*Cassia fistula* Linn	A, B, C, G	2, 3, 9, 43, 63, 64, 113
100.	*Cassia obovata* Sic	A	67
101.	*Cassia occidentalis* Linn	A, I	1, 3, 8, 9, 151, 174, 176
102.	*Cassia tora* Linn	A, B, C	3, 7, 8, 9, 27, 67, 68
103.	*Catharanthus roseus* Don (Syn: *Vinca rosea* Linn)	E	7
104.	*Cedrus deodara* Lond	D, G	3, 7, 9, 21, 28
105.	*Celastrus paniculata* Willd	A, B, C, D, I, J	2, 3, 7, 8, 38, 70-73
106.	*Centella asiatica* Urban	H, J	7
107.	*Centratherum anthelminticum* Ktze	C	27, 38
108.	*Chenopodium album* Linn (Syn: *C. hybridum* Linn)	H	25
109.	*Chenopodium quinoa* Willd	E	7
110.	*Chrozophora prostata* Dalz	H, I	7
111.	*Chrysanthanum balsmitta* Linn	E	1
112.	*Chrysanthanum vulgare* Linn	E	1
113.	*Cichorium intybus* Linn	D, J	7, 28, 74
114.	*Cinnamomum iners* Reinw	C	31
115.	*Cinnamomum zeylanicum* Nees	A, J	7
116.	*Citrus sp*	A, H	25, 76
117.	*Clausena pentaphylla* DC	E, H	7
118.	*Clerodendron phlomides* Linn	D, J	3, 7, 27, 28
119.	*Coccinia indica* Wright & Arn	H	2, 25, 28
120.	*Cocculus pendulus* Diels	C, G	3, 21, 38
121.	*Cocus nucifera* Linn	A, B	2, 3, 7, 27
122.	*Colubrina asiatica* Brongn	A	52
123.	*Commiphora mukul* Hook	D	2, 3, 7, 27, 28
124.	*Conium maculatum* Linn	E	1
125.	*Convolvulus paniculatus* Linn	A,H,J	5,7
126.	*Corchorus aestuans* Linn	G	21, 38
127.	*Corchorus depressus* Christ	A	5
128.	*Corchorus olitorius* Linn	H	25
129.	*Coriandrum sativum* Linn	E, H, J	1, 7
130.	*Corylus avellena* Linn	H	7
131.	*Costus speciosus* Sm	C, D	3, 27, 31
132.	*Crataeva nurvala* Buch-Ham	D	3, 28
133.	*Crocus sativus* Linn	J	7
134.	*Crotolaria burhia* Buch-Ham	G	21, 41
135.	*Crotolaria juncea* Linn	A, B, D, G	3, 77-80
136.	*Crotolaria laburnifolia* Linn	D	3, 28
137.	*Croton sparsiflorus* Morong	A, D	7, 81
138.	*Cucumis melo* Linn	H	7, 25
139.	*Cucumis sativus* Linn	D, H	7, 25
140.	*Cuminum cyminum* Linn	J	7
141.	*Curculigo orchioides* Gaertn	C, G, J	7, 9, 27
142.	*Curcuma longa* Linn	A, B, D, E, F, G, I, J	2, 3, 5, 7, 8, 14, 18, 27, 28, 82-97, 100, 174

(Contd.)

S. No.	Plant	Activities Reported	Reference
143.	*Cuscuta reflexa* Roxb	C, D	27
144.	*Cyamopsis tetragenolobus* Linn	H	7, 25
145.	*Cynodon dactylon* Pers	C	3, 9, 14
146.	*Cyperus compactus* Retz	D,G	21, 41
147.	*Cyperus niveus* Retz	C	3, 9
148.	*Cyperus rotundus* Linn	A, D	3
149.	*Cyperus scariosus* Roxb	D, J	3, 7
150.	*Dalbergia lanceolaria* Linn	D	3, 28
151.	*Dalbergia sissoo* Roxb	A, B, D, E, I	2, 3, 7, 8, 98-100, 176
152.	*Datura metel* Linn	G	3
153.	*Delphinium denudatum* Wall	E	7
154.	*Desmodium gangeticum* DC	A, B, D	3, 28, 184, 185
155.	*Dioscorea pentaphylla* Linn	D	21
156.	*Diospyros chloroxylon* Roxb	C	31
157.	*Diospyros cordifolia* Roxb	D	3, 27, 28
158.	*Diospyros kaki* L.f.	H	25
159.	*Diospyros malabarica* Desr	G	41
160.	*Diospyros marmorata* Parker	C	17
161.	*Diospyros montana* Roxb	A, G	7, 14, 101
162.	*Diospyros peregrina* Gurke	C	3
163.	*Dracocephalium maldavicum* Linn	H	7
164.	*Echinacea purpurea* Moench	E	7
165.	*Eclipta alba* Hassk	A,C,J	3, 7, 9, 102
166.	*Elacia guinensis*	H	7
167.	*Elettaria cardamomum* Mat	A, J	7
168.	*Embelia ribes* Burm f	A, H	2, 7, 103
169.	*Embelia tsjerium-cottam* A.DC	A	103
170.	*Embelia viridiflora* Scheff	D	15
171.	*Emblica officinalis* Gaertn.	A, C, H	3, 7, 9, 25, 104
172.	*Eneste superbum* Cheesm	C	3, 105
173.	*Enicostemma littorale* Blume	A	42
174.	*Eruca sativa* Mill	A, C	3, 8
175.	*Erythra roxburghii* Don	I	2, 8
176.	*Eugenia caryophyllata* Thunb	I	7
177.	*Eulopia campestris* Wall	H, J	7
178.	*Euphorbia hirta* Linn	G, H	3, 9, 25
179.	*Euphorbia pilutifera* Linn	I	2, 8
180.	*Euphorbia prolifera* Ham	G	9
181.	*Euphorbia prostrata* Ait (Syn: *E. thymifolia*)	A, B	3, 68, 69, 174
182.	*Euryale ferox* Salisb	J	7
183.	*Evolvulus alcinoides* Linn	A, B, I, J	2, 7, 8, 106
184.	*Ficus amplissima* Smith	G	41
185.	*Ficus carica* Linn	H	25
186.	*Ficus nemoralis* Wall	G	41
187.	*Ficus religiosa* Linn	A, B, C	2, 7, 27

(Contd.)

S. No.	Plant	Activities Reported	Reference
188.	*Foeniculum vulgare* Mill	H, J	25
189.	*Fumaria officinalis* Linn	H, I, J	7, 27
190.	*Fumaria vailanti* Linn	A	100, 107
191.	*Garcinia morella* Derr	A, B, D, E	27, 108-111, 149, 150
192.	*Garcinia talbotii* Raizada ex Santap	A, C	3, 6
193.	*Gardenia gummifera* Linn	E	7
194.	*Gardenia turgida* Roxb	C, G	9
195.	*Gentiana dahurica* Fisch	I	2, 8
196.	*Geranium pratense* Linn	E	1
197.	*Ginkgo biloba* Linn	J	7
198.	*Glycine max* Merr	H	7, 25
199.	*Glycyrrhiza glabra* Linn	A, D, J	2, 3, 5, 7, 28
200.	*Gmelina arborea* Roxb	C, J	3, 7, 9
201.	*Gmelina asiatica* Linn	G, J	7, 21, 41
202.	*Gmelina philippinensis* Chem	G	41
203.	*Gossypium sp.*	E, H	7, 27
204.	*Grewia hirsuta* Vahl	C	3
205.	*Gymnema sylvestre* Roxb	D, E	2
206.	*Gyrandropsis pentaphylla* DC	G	3
207.	*Hedera helix* Linn	D	7
208.	*Hedychium spicatum* Pouch Hem	D, J	7, 21, 31
209.	*Helianthus annuus* Linn	E	7
210.	*Helleborus niger* Linn	H	7
211.	*Hemidesmus indicus* Roxb	C, D, J	7, 27, 28, 113
212.	*Hibiscus ficulneus* Linn	H	25
213.	*Hibiscus rosa sinensis* Linn	D, H	14, 25, 28
214.	*Hippophae rhamnoides* Linn	E, H	7, 25
215.	*Holarrhena antidysentrica* Wall	G, J	7, 9
216.	*Hydnocarpus laurifolia* Selumer	B	2, 27
217.	*Hydrastis canadensis* Linn	J	7
218.	*Hydrocotyle asiatica* Linn	B, J	7, 27
219.	*Hydychium spicatus* Hamm ex Smith	D	28
220.	*Hyoscymus niger* Linn	J	7
221.	*Hypericum mysorense* Hynae	B	33
222.	*Hypericum perforatum* Linn	E	7
223.	*Illicium verum* Hook	A	114
224.	*Indiqofera aspalathoides* Vahl	E	7
225.	*Indigofera heterantha* Wall	G	9
226.	*Indiqofera mysorensis* Rottl	G	15, 21
227.	*Inula cappa* F Vill	G	21
228.	*Inula racemosa* Hook F	B, D, F	14, 186-188
229.	*Ipomoea aquatica* Forsk	H	25
230.	*Ipomoea dichroa* Choicy	G	21, 41
231.	*Ipomoea digitata* Forsk	J	7

(Contd.)

S. No.	Plant	Activities Reported	Reference
232.	*Ipomoea hederacea* Jacq	I	8, 2
233.	*Ipomea leari* Pext	G	21, 38
234.	*Ipomoea turpethrum* Roxb	D	28, 115
235.	*Jasminum auriculatum* Vahl	E	7
236.	*Jasminum coarctum* Roxb	D	17
237.	*Jasminum dispermum* Wall	G	41
238.	*Jasminum officinale* Linn	G	9
239.	*Jasminum rigidum* Zank	G	15
240.	*Jatropha curcus* Linn	A	5
241.	*Jatropha multifida* Linn	E	7
242.	*Juglans regia* Linn	C, H, J	7, 25, 31
243.	*Juniperus communis* Linn	B	7, 27, 68
244.	*Juniperus squamata* Hem ex Lambert	G	21, 41
245.	*Kalanchae integra* Kuntze	E, G	6, 7, 21
246.	*Lactuca sativa* Linn	H	25
247.	*Lactuca scariola* Linn	I	2, 7, 8
248.	*Lanamelia virginia*	H	7
249.	*Lavandula stoechas* Linn	A, I, J	2, 5, 8, 116
250.	*Lawsonia inermis* Linn	D, H, I, J	2, 7, 8, 186
251.	*Leptadenia reticulata* Hook f	A, B	223
252.	*Levisticum officinale* Koch	E	1
253.	*Lithospermum erythrorhizon* Sieb et Zuc C	E	7
254.	*Litsea chinensis* Lamk	A	16
255.	*Lobelia nicotianaefolia* Heynae	B, C	27
256.	*Lonicera japonica* Thunb	B	7
257.	*Luffa acutangula* Roxb	A	27
258.	*Luffa graveolens* Roxb	G	6, 21
259.	*Macadamia ternifolia* Muell	H	7
260.	*Madhuca butyracea* Roxb	D	28
261.	*Mallotus philippinensis* Muell Arg	A, B	2, 27
262.	*Mallotus stenanthus* Muell Arg	G	21, 31
263.	*Malpighia glabra* Linn	H	25
264.	*Malpighia punicefolia* Linn	H	25
265.	*Matricaria chamomilla* Linn	E	7
266.	*Matricia recutita* Linn	E	1
267.	*Malva rotundifolia* Linn	A	5
268.	*Melaleuca sativa*	J	7
269.	*Melia azadirach* Linn	A, B, E, G, I	2, 7, 8, 21, 27, 174, 186
270.	*Melissa officinalis* Linn	E	7
271.	*Mentha arvensis* Linn	A, B	7, 129
272.	*Mentha longifolia* Linn	E	1
273.	*Mentha spicata* Linn	A,B,E	1, 7
274.	*Mesua ferrea* Linn	D	14, 28
275.	*Mimosa pudica* Linn	C, I	2, 8, 38

(Contd.)

S. No.	Plant	Activities Reported	Reference
276.	*Mimosa tenuiflora* Linn	E	7
277.	*Mimusops elengi* Linn	C, D	27
278.	Mimusops hexandra Roxb	H	25
279.	*Moringa oleifera* Lamk	A, B, C, G, H	8, 21, 25, 41, 130-132, 186
280.	*Moringa pterigosperma* Gaertn	A, C, D	7, 28, 130-132
281.	*Mucuna pruriens* DC	B, E, F, J	7, 14, 27, 186
282.	*Musa pardisiaca* Linn	A	5
283.	*Myristica fragrans* Houff	D, J	1, 2, 7, 14
284.	*Myroxylon pereirae* Kl	H	7
285.	*Myrtus communis* Linn	D	28
286.	*Nardostachys jatamansi* DC	J	2, 7
287.	*Nelumbo nucifera* Gaertn	A, C, H	25, 27
288.	*Nepeta hindostana* Ham	D, I	2, 8, 28, 133, 134
289.	*Nerium indicum* Mill	D	2, 14, 27, 28
290.	*Nerium odorum* Soland	A, G, I	2, 8, 19, 29
291.	*Nigella sativa* Linn	A, G, H	2, 5, 9, 14, 25, 32
292.	*Nymphaea sp*	H, I	5, 7, 25, 26, 186
293.	*Ochrocarpus longifolius* Benth	A, D	28, 39
294.	*Ocimum sanctum* Linn	A, B, C, E, F, H, I, J	7, 8, 10, 25, 27, 51, 118, 128, 135, 137, 138, 174, 186, 189-193, 196-205, 207
295.	*Oenothera biennis* Scop	D, E	7
296.	*Olea ferruginea*	H, I	7
297.	*Olea polygama* Wright	G	15, 21
298.	*Onosma bracteatum* Wall	J	7
299.	*Orchis latefolia* Linn	J	7
300.	*Origanum vulgare* Linn	E	1
301.	*Oxalis acetosella* Linn	H	25
302.	*Oxalis corniculata* Linn	A, H	25, 139
303.	*Paederia foetida* Linn	D, G,	9, 28
304.	*Panax ginseng* Meyer	H	7
305.	*Pandanus tectorius* Sol	B, C	27
306.	*Passiflora foetida* Linn	H	21, 33
307.	*Parsiflora incarnata* Linn	H, J	7
308.	*Parsiflora laurifolia* Linn	G	25
309.	*Pavonia odorata* Willd	J	7
310.	*Pedalium murex* Linn	J	7
311.	*Pelargonium zonale* Linn	E	1
312.	*Petroselinum crispum* Mill	E	1
313.	*Peucedanum officinale* Linn	E	1
314.	*Phaseolus radiatus* Lour (Syn. *P. aureus* Roxb)	D, H	7, 28
315.	*Phoenix dactylifera* Linn	J	7
316.	*Photinia integrifolia* Lindl	C, G	6, 21
317.	*Phylanthus emblica* Linn	B, C, J	7, 25, 27
318.	*Picea abies* Linn	A, E	1, 6

(Contd.)

S. No.	Plant	Activities Reported	Reference
319.	*Picrorrhiza kurroa* Royale ex Benth	A, B	142
320.	*Pinus longifolia* Roxb	E, G	1, 7, 21
321.	*Piper* sp.	A, B, E, J	2, 7, 14, 16, 32, 141, 142
322.	*Pistcia lenticus* Linn	A	7
323.	*Pistca stratiotes* Linn	D, E	2
324.	*Pithecellobium dulce* Benth	D, H	7, 25
325.	*Plantago major* Linn	A	5
326.	*Plantago ovata* Forsck	A	5
327.	*Plectranthus incanus* Link	A	144
328.	*Pluchea lanceolata* Oliver et Heirn	D	28
329.	*Plumbago zeylanica* Linn	A, B, C, H, J	7, 14, 27
330.	*Plumeria acutifolia* Poir	D	28
331.	*Pongamia glabra* Vent	A, B	2, 7, 14, 70
332.	*Pongamia pinnata* Merr	A, E	5, 7
333.	*Populus nigra* Linn	E	1
334.	*Populus tremens* Linn	E	1
335.	*Premna integrifolia* Linn	D	28
336.	*Prunus amygdalus* Stok	A, D, H, I	2, 7, 27, 143
337.	*Prunus avium* Linn	H	25
338.	*Prunus cornuta* Stend	C	31
339.	*Psoralea corylifolia* Linn	A, B, D, I, J	2, 7, 8, 14, 20, 27, 28, 75, 144-147, 174, 186
340.	*Psorpis spicigera* Linn	D	28
341.	*Pterocarpus marsupium* Roxb	A, E	27, 148
342.	*Pterocarpus santalinus* Linn	A, I	1, 2, 7, 8, 27, 171, 181
343.	*Puerarea tuberosa* DC	J	7
344.	*Punica granatum* Linn	A, H, J	5, 7, 25
345.	*Randia dumetorum* Lamk	C	9
346.	*Randia spinosa* Br	A	7
347.	*Rauwolfia serpentina* Benth	D, J	7, 28
348.	*Rheum emodi* Wall	D	8, 27, 174, 176
349.	*Rheum rhaponticum* Linn	H	25
350.	*Rhus chinensis* Mill	D	21
351.	*Rhus parviflora* Roxb	C, G	6, 21
352.	*Rhus succedanea* Linn	C, G, J	2, 7, 9
353.	*Rhus wallichi* Hook	D	21
354.	*Ricinus communis* Linn	D, J	7, 28
355.	*Rosa damascena* Mill	A, B, E	1, 7, 8, 174, 211
356.	*Rosa gallica* Linn	H	25
357.	*Rosa involucrata* Roxb	G	41
358.	*Rosa macrophylla* Lindll	H	25
359.	*Rosmarinus officinalis* Linn	E	1, 7
360.	*Rubia cordifolia* Linn	E, G,	9, 14, 21, 27
361.	*Rubia tinctoria* Linn	B, C, H	7

(Contd.)

S. No.	Plant	Activities Reported	Reference
362.	*Ruscus aculiatus* Linn	D	7
363.	*Saccopetalum tomentosum* Hook	A	32
364.	*Sagittaria sagittaefolia* Linn	D	21, 28
365.	*Salvadora persica* Linn	A, C	27
366.	*Salvia aegyptica* linn	J	7
367.	*Salvia officinalis* Linn	E	1, 7
368.	*Santalum album* Linn	A, B, C, D, I, J	2, 7, 8, 27, 174, 213-216
369.	*Sapindus mukurossi* Gaertn	A	5
370.	*Sapindus trifoliatus* Linn	J	7
371.	*Sapium insigne* Trim	D	28
372.	*Saponaria officinalis* Linn	H	7
373.	*Saraca indica* Linn	J	7
374.	*Sarcostemma brevistigma* Wright & Arn	D	28
375.	*Sarcostemma intermedium* Decne	J	7
376.	*Saussurea lappa* Clarke	A, B, G	2, 14, 27
377.	*Schinopsis balansae* Engl	H	7
378.	*Semecarpus anacardium* Linn	A, C, D, G, J	2, 7, 21, 27, 28, 152, 153
379.	*Serenoa repens* Small	B	7
380.	*Shorea robusta* Gaertn	H	7
381.	*Sida cordifolia* Linn	J	7
382.	*Sida lumidia* Cav	D	28
383.	*Sida rhomofilia* Linn	D	28
384.	*Simmondsia chinensis* Sic	H	7
385.	*Smilex china* Linn	D, H, I	7, 8, 174
386.	*Solanum indicum* Linn	F	27
387.	*Solanum nigrum* Linn	A, D, H	5, 25, 27
388.	*Solanum xanthocarpum* Schrad et Wendl	C, G	9
389.	*Sophora japonicum* Linn	C, H	7
390.	*Sphaeranthus indicus* Kurtz	H, I, J	2, 7, 8, 27, 174, 217
391.	*Stinglia ajanensis*	H	7
392.	*Stingla halopetala*	H	7
393.	*Strebulus asper* Lour	G	21, 38
394.	*Strychnos nux vomica* Linn	J	7
395.	*Swertia chirata* Buch Ham	E, H, I	2, 7, 8, 27, 127, 174, 176
396.	*Symplocos paniculata* Wall	C	9
397.	*Symplocos racemosa* Roxb	A, E	7, 27
398.	*Symplocos thaefolia* Buch Ham	G	9
399.	*Syzygium aromaticum* Merr et Perr	A, J	7
400.	*Syzygium caryophyllifolium* DC	D	15
401.	*Syzygium cumini* Skeels	H	25
402.	*Syzygium lactum* Buch Ham	D	17
403.	*Tamarandus indica* Linn	A, C, E, H	9, 25, 27
404.	*Tamarix gallica* Linn	I, J,	2, 7, 8

(Contd.)

S. No.	Plant	Activities Reported	Reference
405.	*Taraxacum officinale* Weber	B, I	27
406.	*Taxus baccata* Linn	D	28
407.	*Tecoma undulata* G Don	A	225
408.	*Tephrosea candida* DC	G	21, 33
409.	*Tephrosea hirta* Ham	G	41
410.	*Tephrosea purpurea* Pers	A, I, J	2, 7, 8, 27, 49, 71, 155
411.	*Terminalia belerica* Roxb	A, E, G, H	5, 7, 9
412.	*Terminalia chebula* Retz	A, B, C, F, G, I	2, 7, 8, 9, 20, 27, 49, 156, 157, 174, 176
413.	*Terminalia paniculata* Roth	G	21
414.	*Thespesia populnea* Soland ex Correa	A, C, E, G	7, 158
415.	*Thuja occidentalis* Linn	H	7, 159
416.	*Thuja orientalis* Linn	H	25
417.	*Thymus serpyllum* Linn	E, H	1, 25
418.	*Tinospora cordifolia* Miers	A, C, D, E, G, I, J	2, 7, 8, 9, 14, 27, 28, 50, 117, 160-165
419.	*Trachyspermum ammi* Sprague	H	7
420.	*Trianthema decandra* Linn	A	5
421.	*Trianthema portulacastrum* Linn	A, D	5, 28
422.	*Tribulus terrestris* Linn	H, J	7, 25
423.	*Tricholepsis glaberrima* DC	H, I	7
424.	*Trichosanthes dioica* Roxb	H, I, J	2, 7, 8, 25
425.	*Tridex procumbens* Linn	E	7
426.	*Trigonella foenum-graecum* Linn	D, H	7, 25, 27
427.	*Trigonella pubescence* Edgew ex Baker	G	41
428.	*Tylophora indica* Burm	D, J	7, 14
429.	*Typha sp*	B	7
430.	*Ulmaria sp*	H	7
431.	*Urginea indica* Kunth	E, G, H	21, 27
432.	*Urtica dioica* Linn	E	7
433.	*Valeriana wallichii* DC	J	7
434.	*Vanda roxburghii* Br	C, D, G	21, 27
435.	*Vanda spathulata* Spreng	C	33
436.	*Vateria indica* Linn	A	32
437.	*Veronica cinerea* Lers	C, E, G	9, 27
438.	*Vetiveria zizanoides* Nash	E, M	7
439.	*Viola tricolor* Linn	E	7
440.	*Vitis vinifera* Linn	J	7
441.	*Withania coagulans* Dunal	D	28
442.	*Withania somnifera* Dunal	B, C, D, J	2, 7, 14, 27, 28
443.	*Zanthoxylum acanthopopium* DC	H	7
444.	*Zanthoxylum alatum* Roxb	A	16
445.	*Zanthoxylum budrunga* Wall	D	28
446.	*Zea mays* Linn	H	7

(Contd.)

S. No.	Plant	Activities Reported	Reference
447.	*Zingiber capitalatum* Roxb	G	15, 21
448.	*Zingiber officinale* Rosc	A, H, J	7, 14, 25
449.	*Zingiber zerumbet* Rosc	A	166, 174, 176
450.	*Zizyphus glaberrima* Santapan	C	31
451.	*Zizyphus jujuba* Lamk	H, I, J	7
452.	*Zizyphus mauritiana* Lamk	H	25
453.	*Zizyphus oenoplia* Mill	A	167
454.	*Zizyphus rugosa* Lamk	C, G	17, 21
455.	*Zizyphus vulgaris* Lamk	A, I	2, 168

Table 4.2 Frequency distribution of activities reported in medicinal plants

Number of Activities	Number of Plants (%)
1	253 (55.84)
2	114 (25.16)
3	53 (11.69)
4	17 (3.75)
5	7 (1.54)
6	6 (1.32)
7	2 (0.44)
8	1 (0.22)

Table 4.3 Frequency distribution of relevant pharmacological activities in plants useful for skin diseases

Pharmacological Activity	Number of Plants (%)
Antibacterial	125 (27.59) ⎤
Antifungal	63 (13.90) ⎬ Antimicrobial
Antiviral	83 (18.32) ⎦ (59.82)
Antiinflammatory	92 (20.30)
Wound Healing	62 (13.68)
Antiallergic/Antihistaminic	5 (1.10)
Anticancer	94 (20.75)
Vitamin A,C,E containing	114 (25.16)
Blood Purifying	45 (9.93)
Adaptogenic/Antiageing	88 (19.42)

4.2 HERBO-MINERAL APPROACH

We have always felt that medicine, as it is practiced today, lacks definite objectives and its principles need a thorough review. The basis of treatment is weak, the laws have not been properly codified and the approach is not holistic. These problems were discussed in an earlier publication[169]. Traditional medicinal concepts are based on a harmonius balance of elements, humours and temperaments. Jamia Hamdard and its erstwhile constituent unit, Institute of History of Medicine and Medical Research, has done some pioneering work towards the study of ancient philosophical ideas relating to elements in the light of modern scientific knowledge and organized four International Conferences at New Delhi (1983), Karachi (1987), Ankara (1989) and again at New Delhi (1993). This led to emergence and development of Medical Elementology as a new discipline in science.

We proposed a quadrilateral approach:

i. Elemental composition of human body in healthy subjects.

ii. Changes in elemental composition in different diseases.

iii. Determination of elements in simple and compound drugs.

iv. Changes in body elements through the use of these drugs leading to restoration of health[170].

The first two aspects have received considerable attention in recent years with voluminous data available from all parts of the world. Normal human values for elemental content in the whole body and in different tissues and body fluids were compiled by Iyengar and co-workers[171]. The association of component elements with various human diseases and aging was reviewed by us[172,173]. A lot remains to be done on the remaining two aspects. We are aware that the four facets of the proposed quadrilateral approach, though easily enumerated, are very difficult in application. At the present state of knowledge, there appear to be two major hurdles: (a) wide variations in base line values, and (b) lack of precision analytical techniques which are practicable in field conditions. But a beginning has to be made. This study is an attempt towards the third aspect viz. elemental composition of the simple drugs. Since herbal products constitute the bulk of materia medica of Indian systems of medicine, we start with medicinal plants with a therapeutic potential in skin diseases. Vast experience (treated more than 5 million patients over a period of about 60 years) of one of us (Abdul Hameed) helped in preparing a priority list of plants investigations on which are likely to be more rewarding (Table 4.4).

Table 4.4 Priority list of plants selected for studying therapeutic value in skin diseases

S. No.	Botanical Name	Unani Name
1.	*Acacia arabica*	KIKAR
2.	*Albizzia lebbeck*	SIRAS
3.	*Aloe vera*	GHEEKANWAR
4.	*Ammi majus*	ATRILAL
5.	*Artemisia absinthum*	AFSANTEEN ROOMI
6.	*Azadirachta indica*	NIM
7.	*Bauhinia variegata*	KACHNAL
8.	*Berberis aristata*	DARHALD

(Contd.)

S. No.	Botanical Name	Unani Name
9.	*Cassia absus*	CHAKSU
10.	*Cassia angustifolia*	SENNA
11.	*Cassica occidentalis*	KASONDI
12.	*Curcuma longa*	HALDI
13.	*Dalbergia sissoo*	SHISHAM
14.	*Daphne mezerium*	MARZIUN
15.	*Desmodium gangeticum*	SHALWAM
16.	*Euphorbia thymifolia*	CHOTI DUDHI
17.	*Fumaria indica*	SHAHTARA
18.	*Inula racemosa*	RASAN
19.	*Lawsonia alba*	HINA
20.	*Melia azadarach*	BAKAIN
21.	*Moringa oleigera*	SONJANA
22.	*Mucuna pruriens*	KONCH
23.	*Nymphaea alba*	NILOFAR
24.	*Ocimum sanctum*	TULSI
25.	*Plumbago rosea*	LAL CHITRA
26.	*Psoralea corylifolia*	BABCHI
27.	*Pterocarpus santalinus*	SANDAL SURKH
28.	*Rheum emodi*	REVAND CHINI
29.	*Rosa domascena*	GULAB
30.	*Rumex maritimus*	JANGLI PALAK
31.	*Santalum album*	SANDAL SAFED
32.	*Smilex china*	CHOBCHINI
33.	*Sphaeranthus indicus*	MUNDI
34.	*Swertia chirata*	CHIRATA
35.	*Terminalia chbula*	HALEELA
36.	*Thevetia nerifolia*	PILA KANER
37.	*Tinospora cordifolia*	GILOE
38.	*Wrightia tinctoria*	INDRAJOU SHIREEN
39.	*Zingiber zerumbet*	NARKACHOOR

4.3 SHORT MONOGRAPHS ON SOME PLANTS USED IN SKIN DISEASES AND THEIR ELEMENTAL COMPOSITION

The following pages describe these plants in detail along with their photograp'

SCIENTIFIC NAME	:	*Acacia arabica* Willd
UNANI NAME	:	KIKAR/BABOOL
FAMILY	:	*Mimosaceae*
PARTS USED	:	Bark, gum, leaves, seeds and pods

PHARMACOLOGICAL PROPERTIES RELEVANT TO THERAPEUTIC USE IN SKIN DISEASES

It is attributed with antiseptic, blood purifying, astringent, styptic and demulcent properties. The plant is rich in tannin content[3,8,174,175]. Other species of *Acacia* are reported to elicit interesting biological effects e.g. antibacterial and antifungal activity in *A. catechu*[11] and *A. ruguta*[180] and antiinflammatory effects in *A. farnesiana*[181]. Another species of this genera viz. *Acacia auriculiformis* was shown to possess antiviral activity in screening programme at the Central Drug Research Institute, Lucknow[14,21].

ELEMENTAL COMPOSITION[176]

Element	Concentration (mg/g ash)
Magnesium	2.19
Calcium	978.70
Lead	0.12
Copper	0.05
Mercury	ND
Cobalt	ND
Zinc	0.26
Iron	0.02
Chromium	ND
Cadmium	ND
Manganese	0.07
Nickel	ND
Silver	ND
Molybdenum	ND

ND : Not detected

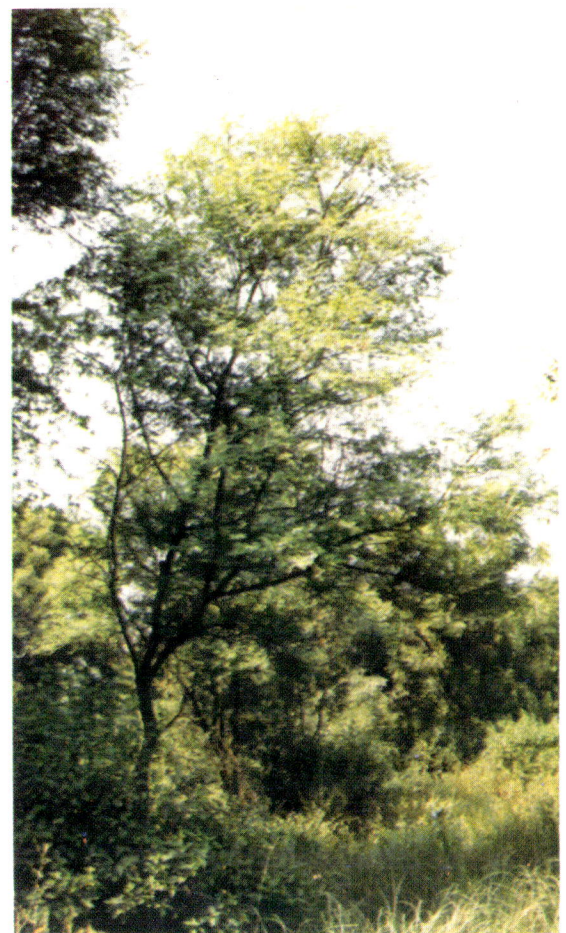
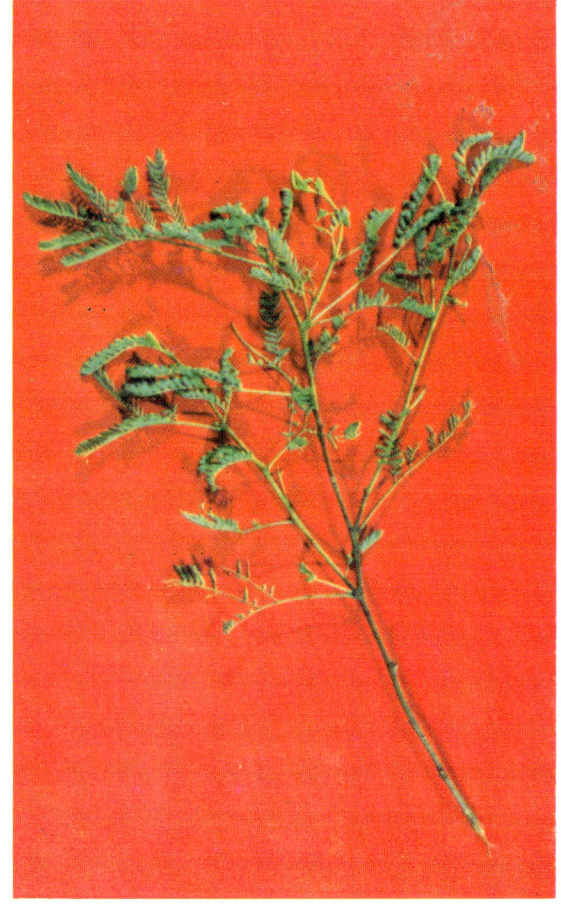

Acacia arabica

(Field Photo : Dr. M.P. Sharma and Mr. Kaiser N. Khan)

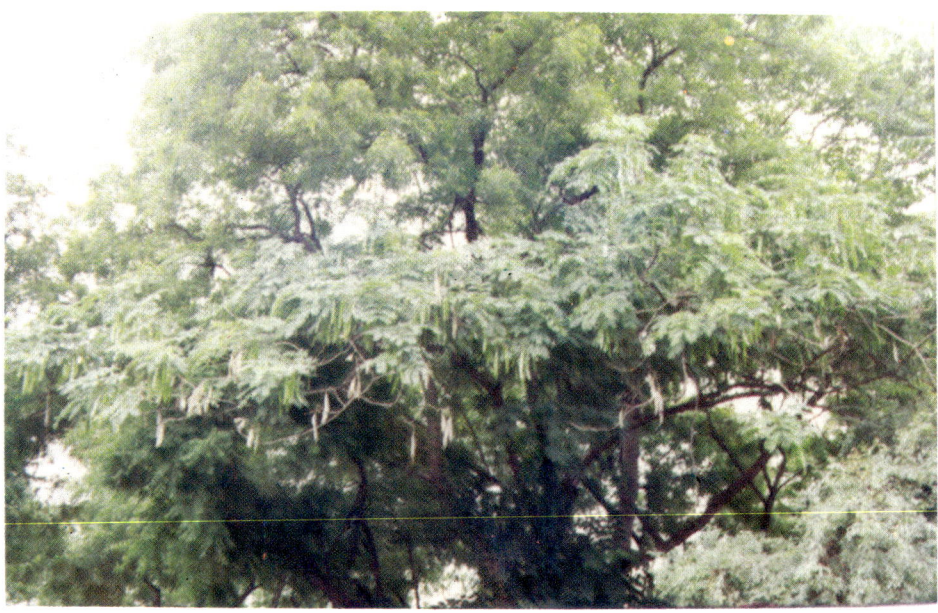

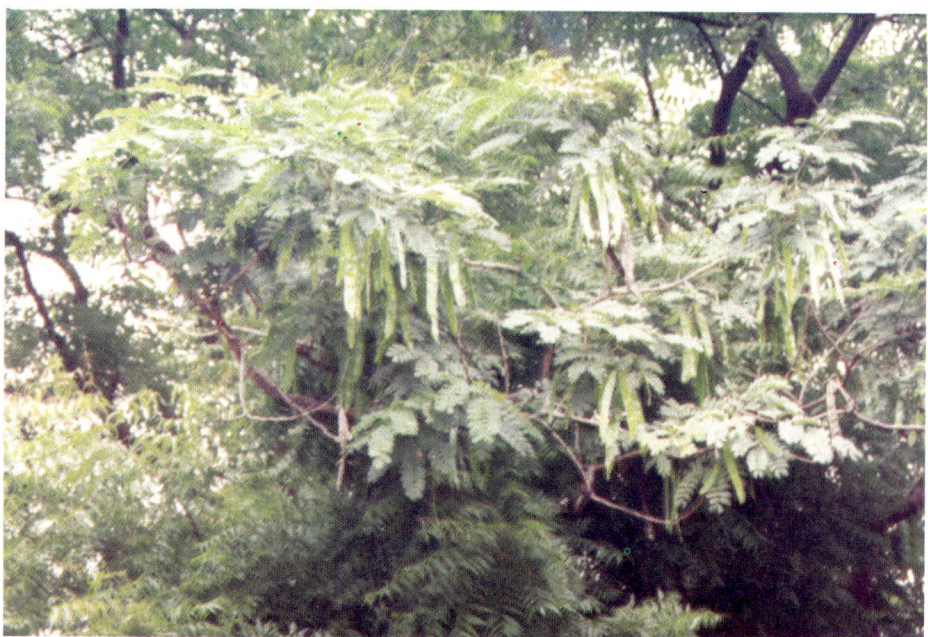

Albizzia lebbeck
(Field Photo : Dr. M.P. Sharma and Mr. Kaiser N. Khan)

SCIENTIFIC NAME	:	*Albizzia lebbeck* Benth
UNANI NAME	:	SIRAS
FAMILY	:	*Leguminosae*
PARTS USED	:	Bark seeds and leaves

PHARMACOLOGICAL PROPERTIES RELEVANT TO THERAPEUTIC USE IN SKIN DISEASES

The plant is reputed for its antiseptic, blood purifying, antitubercular, antiinflammatory and detoxicant effects and usefulness in leprosy[3,8,174]. Tissue culture studies at CDRI, Lucknow revealed anticancer activity against human epidermal carcinoma of the naropharynx[9]. The plant is also reported to possess anti-allergic and immunomodulating effects. It elicited significant chromoglycate like action on mast cells, inhibited PHA-induced blastogenic response of human lymphocytes in sensitized guinea pigs, markedly reduced the secretion of macrophage migration inhibitor and protected sensitized guinea pigs against horse serum antigen[14].

ELEMENTAL COMPOSITION OF LEAVES[227,228]

Element	Concentration (mg/g ash)
Copper	0.117
Zinc	0.211
Iron	0.430
Manganese	0.355
Magnesium	60.600
Chromium	0.117
Nickel	0.013
Cadmium	0.0008
Cobalt	0.006
Lead	0.005
Silver	0.002
Molybdenum	0.005
Tin	0.0001

ND : Not detected

SCIENTIFIC NAME	:	*Aloe vera* Linn
Synonym	:	*Aloe barbadensis* Mill
UNANI NAME	:	GHEEKANWAR
FAMILY	:	*Liliaceae*
PARTS USED	:	Whole plant or leaves in the form of pulp or juice

PHARMACOLOGICAL PROPERTIES RELEVANT TO THERAPEUTIC USE IN SKIN DISEASES

Transeverse cuts are given on large fleshy leaves to drain out and collect thick juice. The latter darkens on storage or boiling yielding the commercial drug aloes (*musabbar*) in the form of dark hard material. External application of the mucilage or the preserved drug as such or in the form of a poultice is useful in inflammatory conditions and itching of the skin. The drug contains a mixture of glycosides called 'alloin'. The principal constituent is barbaloin (a water soluble glycoside). Other constituents include isobarbaloin, b-barbaloin, aloe emodin, resins etc[174]. The plant is attributed with blood purifying properties in Unani medicine[8]. A vaseline based ointment of the expressed juice has been reported to hasten healing of wounds (thermal burns and radiation injury) in albino rats. Hydroxyproline and mucopolysaccharide contents were significantly increased in treated animals[177].

ELEMENTAL COMPOSITION[227,228]

Element	Concentration (mg/g ash)
Copper	0.062
Zinc	0.015
Iron	2.060
Manganese	0.084
Magnesium	41.300
Chromium	0.019
Nickel	0.008
Cadmium	0.0004
Cobalt	0.007
Lead	0.001
Silver	0.002
Molybdenum	0.004
Tin	0.0001

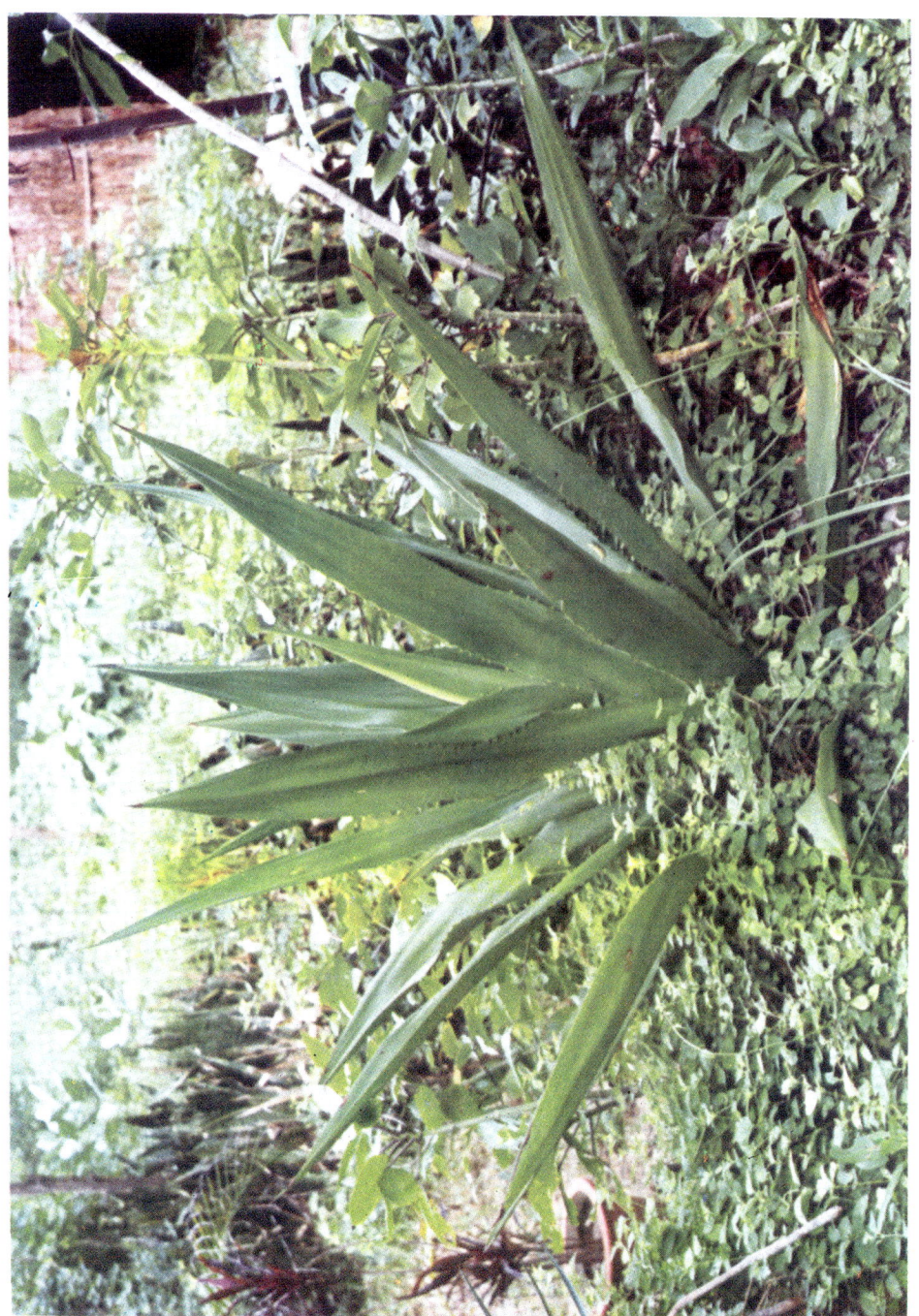

Aloe vera

(Field Photo : Dr. M.P. Sharma and Mr. Kaiser N. Khan)

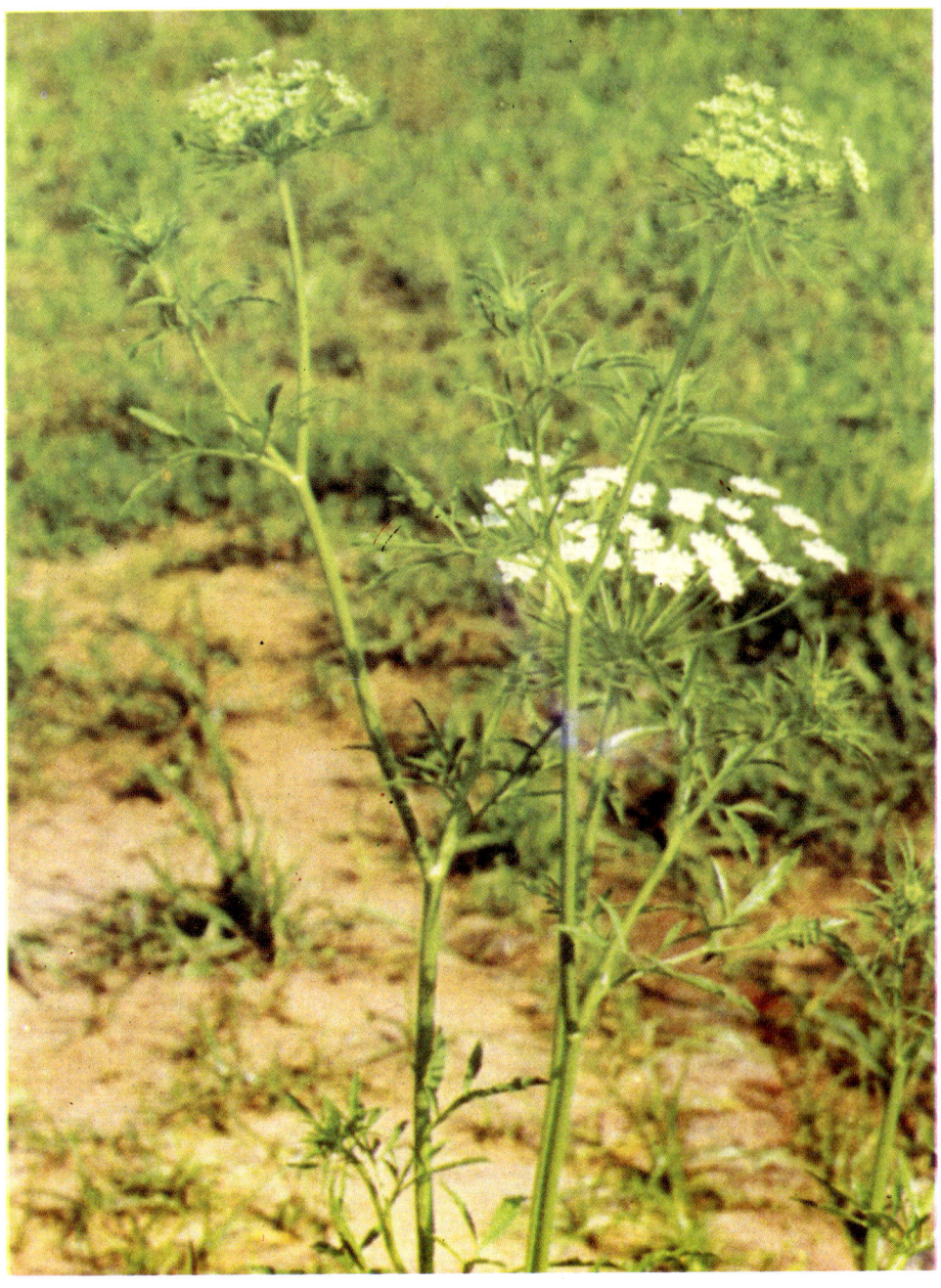

Ammi majus

(Field Photo : Dr. S. Raisuddin)

SCIENTIFIC NAME	:	*Ammi majus* Linn
UNANI NAME	:	BABCHI
FAMILY	:	*Umbelliferae*
PARTS USED	:	Fruits and seeds

PHARMACOLOGICAL PROPERTIES RELEVANT TO THERAPEUTIC USE IN SKIN DISEASES

Egyptians have a long tradition of the use of this plant for the treatment of leucoderma. Studies during the last three decades have confirmed its efficacy in this disease. The plant has been extensively investigated for various aspects including cultivation, chemical, pharmacological, toxicological and clinical investigations. Some details on its history, chemistry, clinical efficacy, possible mechanism of action and toxicity are given in Chapter 6 (please see Section 6.4.1).

ELEMENTAL COMPOSITION[227,228]

Element	Concentration (mg/g ash)
Copper	1.150
Zinc	0.065
Iron	0.130
Manganese	0.024
Magnesium	2.800
Chromium	0.002
Nickel	0.032
Cadmium	0.0004
Cobalt	0.007
Lead	0.150
Silver	0.001
Molybdenum	0.006
Tin	0.0001

SCIENTIFIC NAME	:	*Artemisia absinthum* Linn
UNANI NAME	:	AFSANTEEN ROOMI
FAMILY	:	*Compositae*
PARTS USED	:	Whole plant

PHARMACOLOGICAL PROPERTIES RELEVANT TO THERAPEUTIC USE IN SKIN DISEASES

The essential oil contains absinthin (a bitter glycoside), thujone and thujyl alcohol. The drug, though chiefly used as an anthelmintic, possesses antiseptic properties with beneficial effect in cutaneous ailments, burns, wounds and dropsy[8,174]. Ethanolic extract of another species *A. scoparia* is reported to elicit antibacterial effects *in vitro*[5].

ELEMENTAL COMPOSITION[227,228]

Element	Concentration (mg/g ash)
Copper	0.103
Zinc	0.219
Iron	23.000
Manganese	0.425
Magnesium	67.000
Chrcmium	0.026
Nickel	0.064
Cadmium	0.0003
Cobalt	0.018
Lead	0.850
Silver	0.002
Molybdenum	0.029
Tin	0.0001

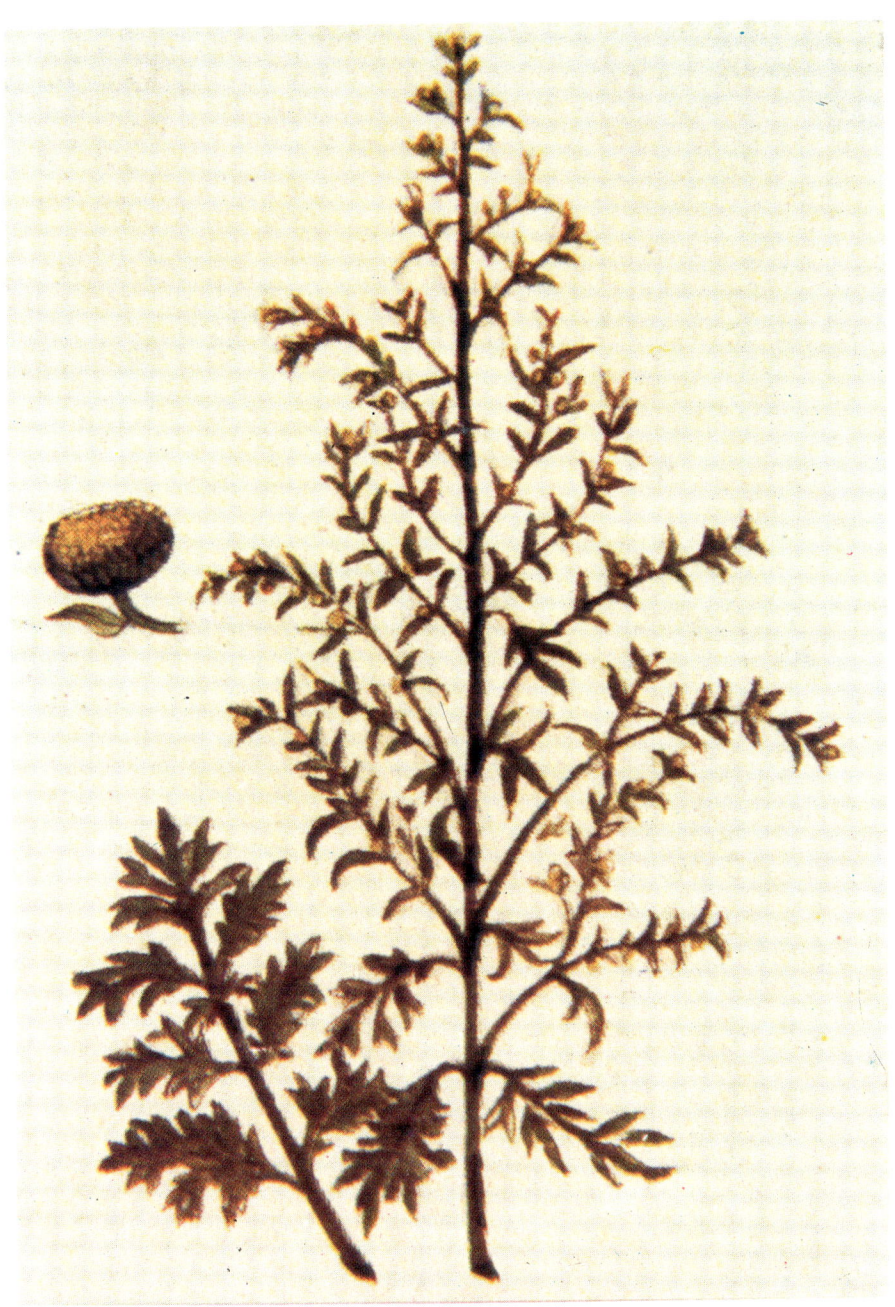

Artemisia absinthum

(Courtesy : Hamdard Dawakhana, Delhi)

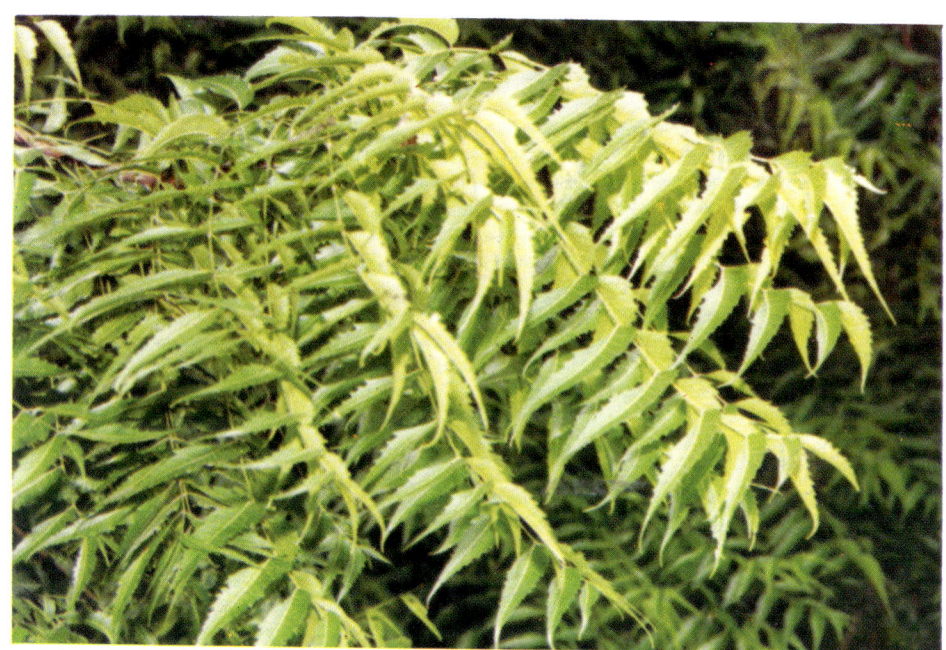

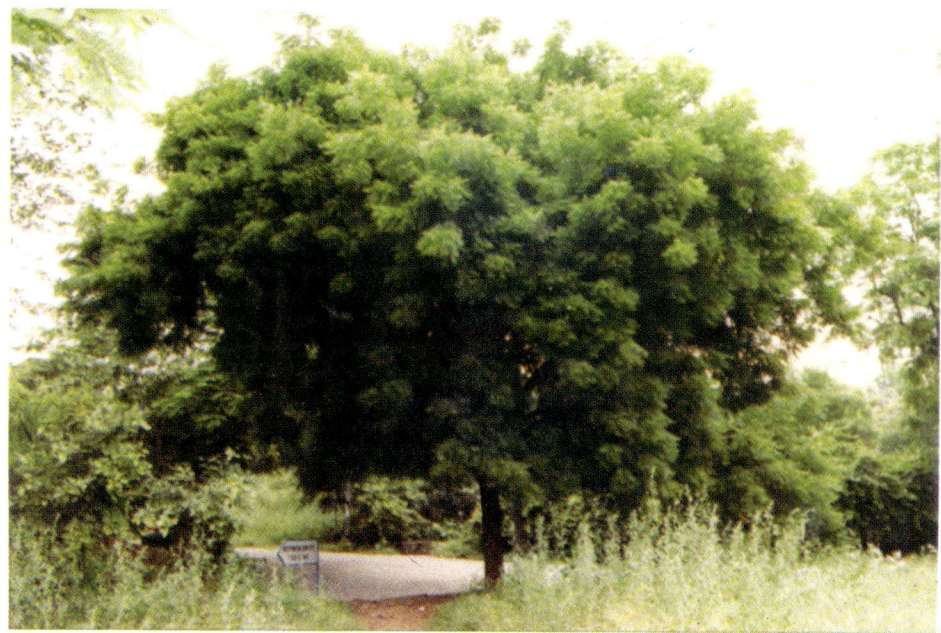

Azadirachta indica

(Field Photo : Dr. M.P. Sharma and Mr. Kaiser N. Khan)

SCIENTIFIC NAME	:	*Azadirachta indica* A Juss
Synonym	:	Melia azadirachta Linn
UNANI NAME	:	NIM
FAMILY	:	*Meliaceae*
PARTS USED	:	Leaves, tender stem, bark, young fruits

PHARMACOLOGICAL PROPERTIES RELEVANT TO THERAPEUTIC USE IN SKIN DISEASES

Margosa oil is highly reputed for its antimicrobial effects. Essential oil from leaves, seeds and bark is reported to elicit antibacterial (against gram positive and gram negative organisms), antitubercular (even against streptomycin resistant strains), antifungal and antiviral effects. This was demonstrated both by *in vitro* and *in vivo* studies[3,7,8,14,21,42,44,45]. Rao and coworkers[178] subjected 200 clinical isolates of bacteria to in vitro antibacterial effects of neem oil and found 92% of these isolates to be susceptible. Minimum inhibitory concentrations ranged between 1:4 to 1:64 dilutions of the oil. Decoction of bark and seeds, nimbin, nimbidin and sodium nimbinate isolated from the oil revealed antiinflammatory effects against carrageenin induced edema, formalin induced arthritis and granuloma pouch formed by croton oil[3,28]. The plant extracts or purified principles are incorporated in many traditional blood purifying formulations, ointments, soaps, creams, lotions, tooth pastes and other cosmetics for use in treatment of acne, pimples, boils, scabies, dermatitis, frunculosis, herpes, bleeding gums, pyrrhoea, healing of wounds, burns, ulcers and for the improvement of complexion[3,7].

ELEMENTAL COMPOSITION:[176,179]

Element	Concentration (mg/g ash)	
	Bark	Leaves
Magnesium	16.96	0.95
Calcium	962.08	—
Lead	0.19	0.06
Copper	0.04	0.01
Mercury	ND	ND
Cobalt	Traces	0.002
Zinc	0.23	0.03
Iron	0.19	0.29
Chromium	ND	0.001
Cadmium	Traces	ND
Manganese	0.11	0.04
Nickel	ND	ND
Silver	ND	ND
Molybdenum	ND	ND
Phosphorus	—	0.09
Sodium	—	13.00
Potassium	—	19.00

— Not analysed   ND : Not detected

The oil is reported to contain 0.427 percent sulphur. The germicidal effects of the plant may be partly attributed to its high S content and nimbidal[3].

SCIENTIFIC NAME	:	*Bauhinia variegata* Linn
UNANI NAME	:	KACHNAL
FAMILY	:	*Caesalpiniaceae*
PARTS USED	:	Bark, Gum, flowers, seeds and root

PHARMACOLOGICAL PROPERTIES RELEVANT TO THERAPEUTIC USE IN SKIN DISEASES

Various parts of the plant possess alterative, astringent and tonic properties. It is incorporated in Unani formulations and used as a blood purifier for the treatment of various skin diseases. Tissue culture studies carried out at the Central Drug Research Institute, Lucknow using the ethanolic extract of stem bark of another species of *Bauhinia* (*B. racemosa*) revealed anticancer activity against human epidermal carcinoma of the nasopharynx[3].

ELEMENTAL COMPOSITION[176]

Element	Concentration (mg/g ash)
Magnesium	2.33
Calcium	959.08
Lead	0.14
Copper	0.03
Mercury	ND
Cobalt	ND
Zinc	0.13
Iron	0.06
Chromium	ND
Cadmium	Traces
Manganese	0.02
Nickel	ND
Silver	ND
Molybdenum	ND

ND : Not detected

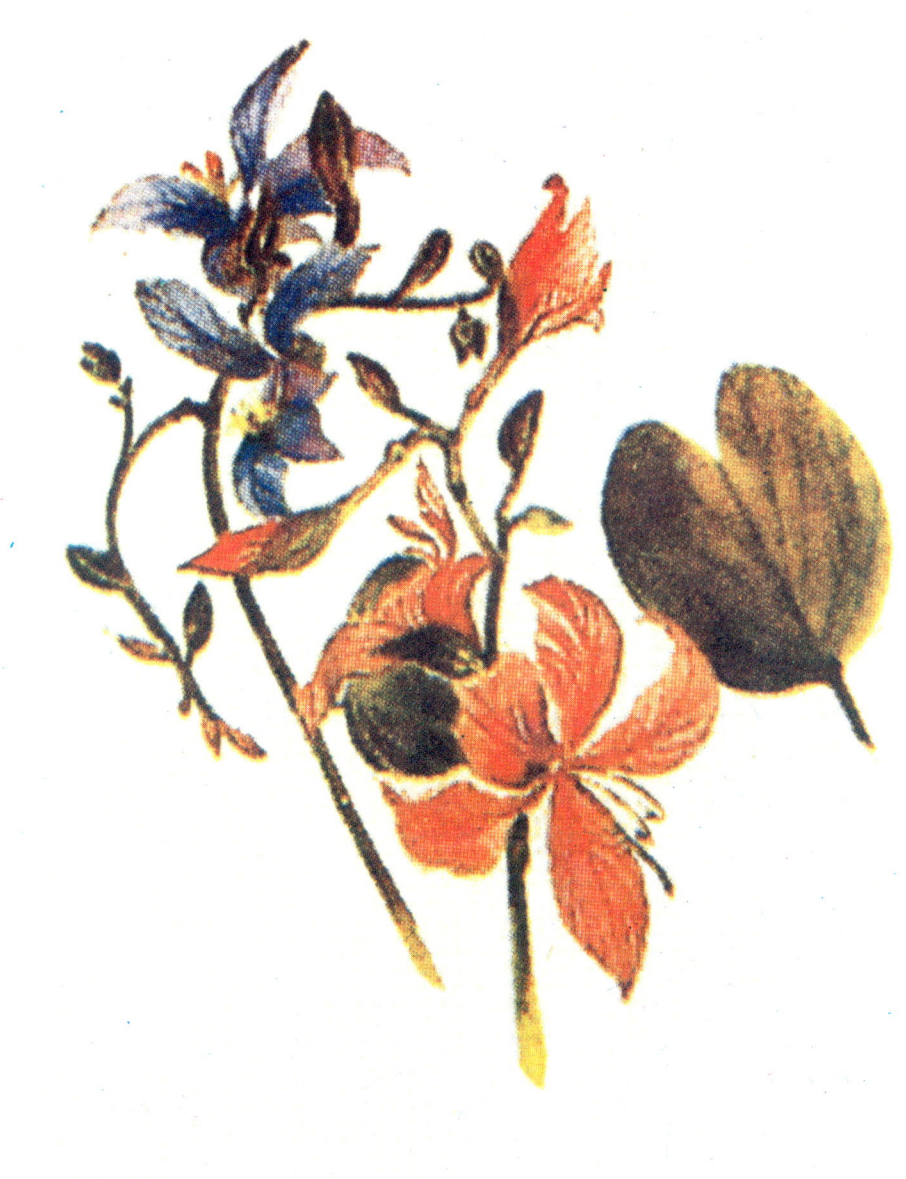

Bauhinia variegata
(Courtesy : Hamdard Dawakhana, Delhi)

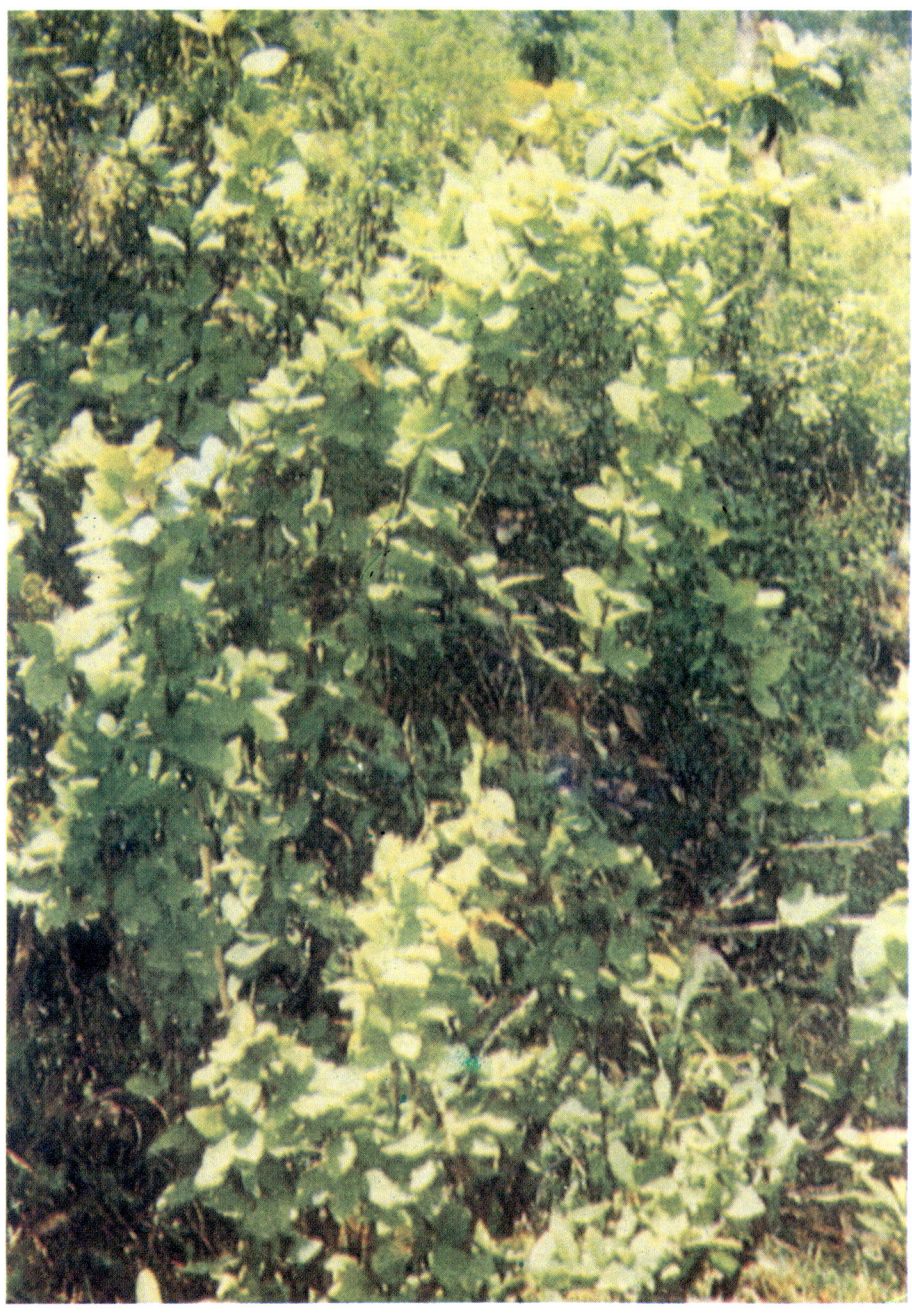

Berberis aristata

(Courtesy : CCRUM, New Delhi)

SCIENTIFIC NAME	:	*Berberis aristata* DC
UNANI NAME	:	DARHALD, RASAUT
FAMILY	:	*Berberidaceae*
PARTS USED	:	Fruit, stem, root bark

PHARMACOLOGICAL PROPERTIES RELEVANT TO THERAPEUTIC USE IN SKIN DISEASES

Berberine bearing plants are reputed for blood purifying properties and for the treatment of skin diseases including its successful therapeutic use in cutaneous leishmaniasis or oriental sore[8,174]. Root bark of *B. aristata* is rich in alkaloidal content and is an official drug of the Indian Pharmacopoeia. The plant is reported to possess antibacterial, antiviral, amoebicidal, antiinflammatory and anticancer properties[3,28]. Berberine sulphate was shown to elicit antimicrobial activity against a wide variety of microorganisms including gram positive and gram negative bacteria, fungi and protozoa. This was attributed to an inhibitory effect of the drug on RNA and protein synthesis[48].

ELEMENTAL COMPOSITION[227,228]

Element	Concentration (mg/g ash)
Copper	0.154
Zinc	0.013
Iron	0.650
Manganese	0.027
Magnesium	1.800
Chromium	0.018
Nickel	0.097
Cadmium	0.0007
Cobalt	0.012
Lead	0.340
Silver	0.005
Molybdenum	0.004
Tin	0.0001

SCIENTIFIC NAME	:	*Cassia absus* Linn
UNANI NAME	:	CHAKSU
FAMILY	:	*Leguminosae*
PARTS USED	:	Leaves and seeds bark

PHARMACOLOGICAL PROPERTIES RELEVANT TO THERAPEUTIC USE IN SKIN DISEASES

Local application of leaves is claimed to heal ulcers, cure leucoderma and elicit beneficial effects in diseases of eye and haemorrhoids[174]. The seeds are attributed with astringent properties and utility in skin and eye affections[3]. Ethanolic extract was reported to inhibit carrageenin induced edema and croton oil induced granuloma in rats indicating its antiinflammatory action[28]. Its alkaloidal principle possesses antibacterial properties[182].

ELEMENTAL COMPOSITION[228]

Element	Concentration (mg/g ash)
Copper	0.221
Zinc	0.360
Iron	85.000
Manganese	0.286
Magnesium	76.000
Chromium	0.009
Nickel	0.025
Cadmium	0.001
Cobalt	0.007
Lead	0.410
Silver	0.001
Molybdenum	0.063
Tin	0.0001

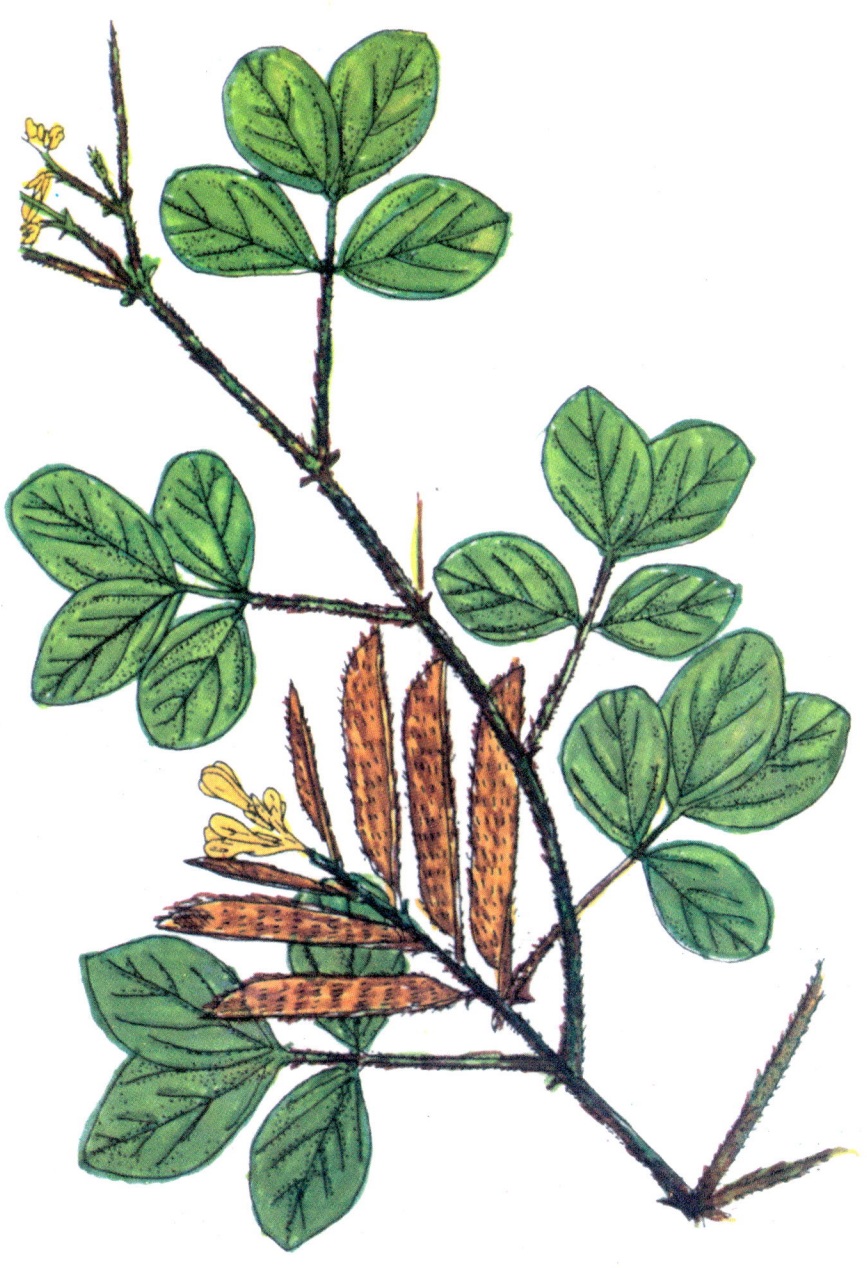

Cassia absus

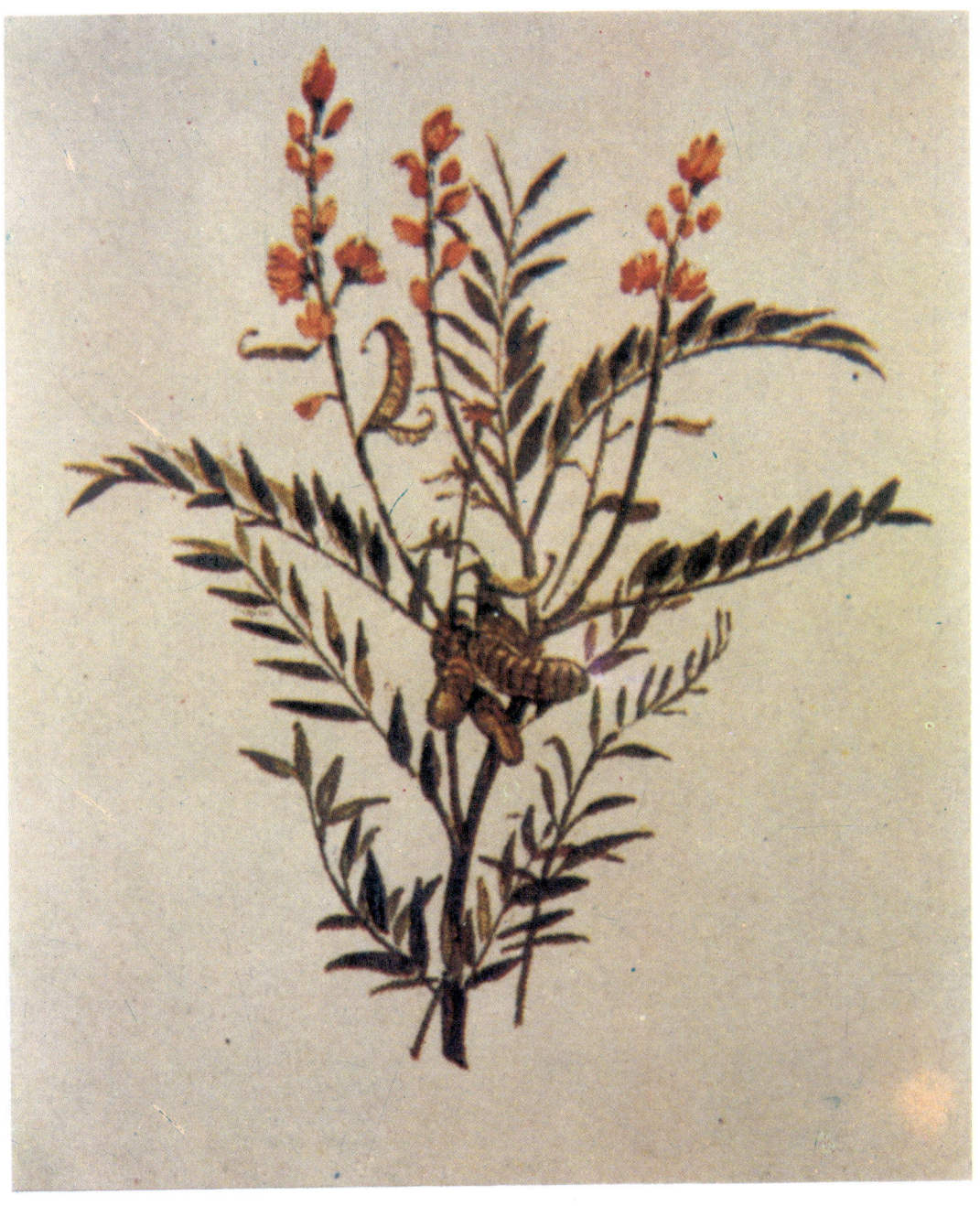

Cassia angustifolia
(Courtesy : Hamdard Dawakhana, Delhi)

SCIENTIFIC NAME	:	*Cassia angustifolia* Vahl
UNANI NAME	:	SENNA
FAMILY	:	*Leguminosae*
PARTS USED	:	Leaves and fruits

PHARMACOLOGICAL PROPERTIES RELEVANT TO THERAPEUTIC USE IN SKIN DISEASES

This drug was known to Arabs since ancient times and was introduced into medicine by them. The drug is claimed to possess cathartic, antimicrobial and antiinflammatory properties and is incorporated in a Unani formulation for blood purifying effects in skin diseases[2,3,8,100,174,176]. The efficacy of *Cassia* species in skin diseases may be attributed to the presence of anthraquinone derivatives (especially chrysophanol) which are the active constituents of Goa powder: a popular remedy for skin diseases[3]. Antifungal and antiinflammatory properties were confirmed in many species of *Cassia* by *in vivo* studies[28,68].

ELEMENTAL COMPOSITION OF LEAVES[176]

Element	Concentration (mg/g ash)
Magnesium	60.631
Calcium	830.564
Lead	0.564
Copper	0.058
Mercury	0.166
Cobalt	ND
Zinc	0.809
Iron	0.112
Chromium	ND
Cadmium	Traces
Manganese	0.207
Nickel	ND
Silver	ND
Molybdenum	ND

ND : Not detected

SCIENTIFIC NAME	:	*Cassia occidentalis* Linn
UNANI NAME	:	KASONDI
FAMILY	:	*Leguminosae*
PARTS USED	:	Leaves and seeds

PHARMACOLOGICAL PROPERTIES RELEVANT TO THERAPEUTIC USE IN SKIN DISEASES

Seeds and leaves possess astringent, antimicrobial and blood purifying properties and are claimed to be of value in skin diseases[1,8,174,176]. Crude extracts, essential oil and anthraquinone derivatives exhibited antibacterial activity[3]. Anthelmintic activity was reported in petroleum ether, chloroform and methanol extracts of seeds and leaves[183].

ELEMENTAL COMPOSITION[228]

Element	Concentration (mg/g ash)
Sodium	2.930
Potassium	22.130
Cadmium	ND
Magnesium	29.140
Manganese	0.320
Iron	0.268
Nickel	0.020
Lead	0.190
Zinc	0.500
Copper	0.200
Chromium	0.090
Cobalt	0.011
Lead	0.610
Silver	0.002
Molybdenum	0.045
Tin	0.0003

ND : Not detected

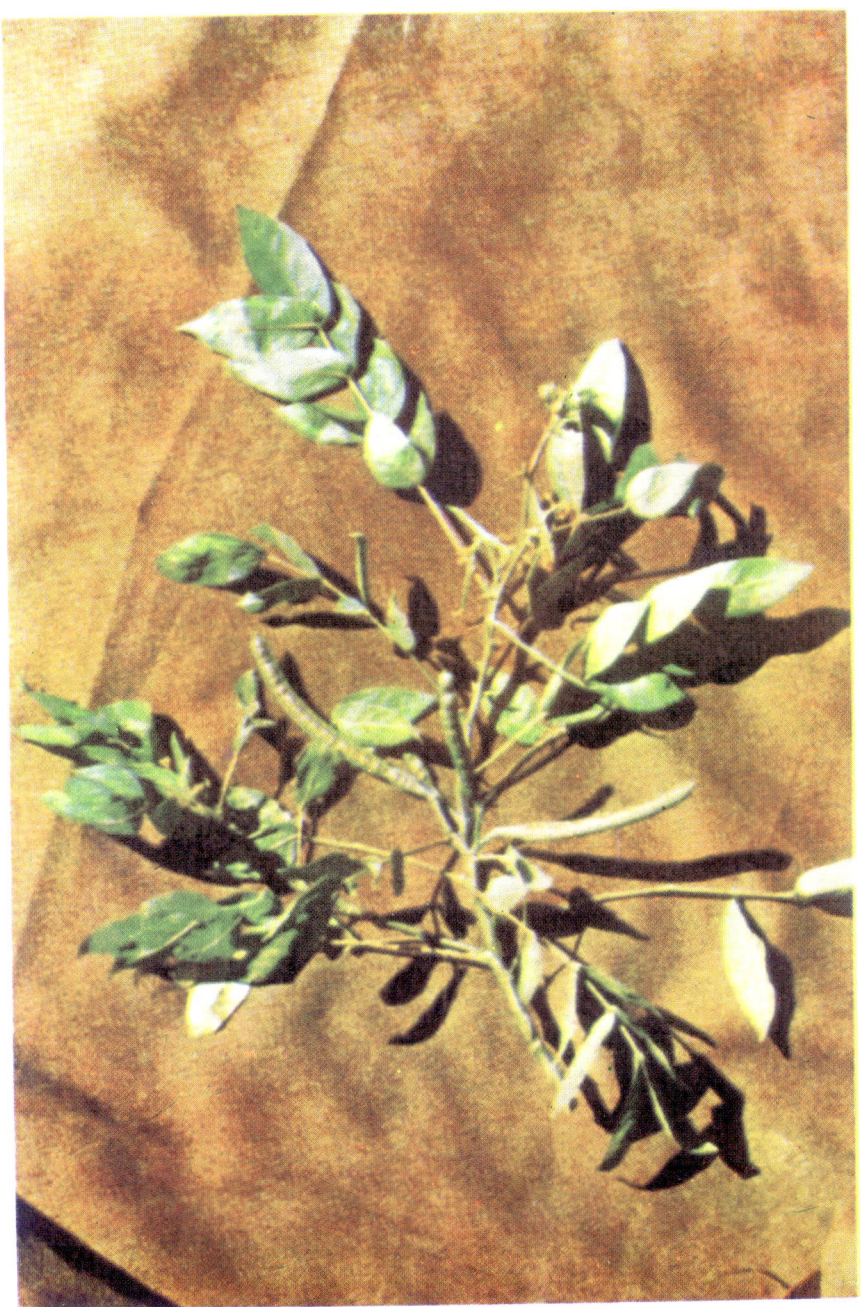

Cassia occidentalis

(Courtesy : Hamdard Dawakhana, Delhi)

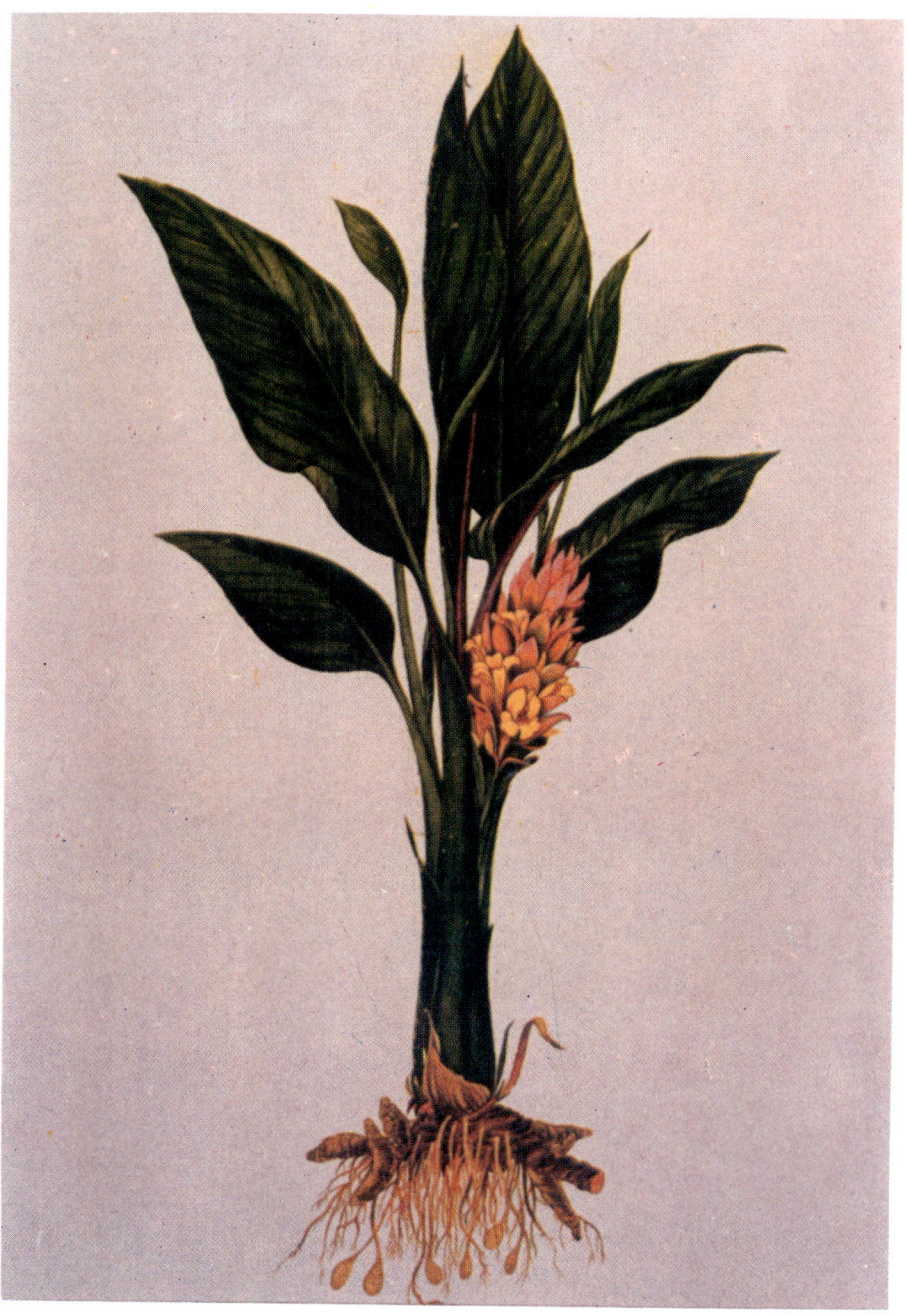

Curcuma longa
(Courtesy : HNF, Delhi)

SCIENTIFIC NAME	:	*Curcuma longa* Linn
UNANI NAME	:	HALDI
FAMILY	:	*Zingiberaceae*
PARTS USED	:	Rhizomes

PHARMACOLOGICAL PROPERTIES RELEVANT TO THE THERAPEUTIC USE IN SKIN DISEASES

It is attributed with blood purifying, antimicrobial, anthelmintic, antiinflammatory, antiulcer, anti-cancer and wound healing properties[18,28,100,174]. Fresh juice of rhizomes or paste prepared from its decoction is often used for local application for soothing effect on inflamed parts and to promote healing. Turmeric mixed with warm milk is a household remedy in India for such effects[174]. Among its varied medicinal properties, the most important is anti-inflammatory action which has been confirmed both by experimental and clinical studies[3,28]. Antiinflammatory effects were reported in crude extracts (ethanol, petroleum ether, water) volatile oil, fractions from the petroleum ether extract, curcumin, sodium curcuminate, and feruloyl-cis 4 hydroxy cinnamoyl methane. The activity was confirmed by a variety of experimental models including edema induced by formalin, Freund's adjuvant and talc, granuloma induced by croton oil and cotton pellet, effect in adrenalectomised animals, and biochemical investigations pertaining to antitrycain, anti-hyaluronidase and prostaglandin activities[86-93]. The anti-inflammatory effects compared well with hydrocortisone and phenylbutazone[3]. Clinical studies revealed hypocholesterolemic action and beneficial effects in inflammatory conditions of the respiratory tract[3,82,95]. Crude extracts exhibited antibacterial effects particularly against gram positive organisms[5,84]. Antifungal activity was observed in the essential oil of rhizomes[83].

ELEMENTAL COMPOSITION[210]

Element	Concentration (mg/g ash)
Sodium	6.360
Potassium	54.470
Calcium	0.065
Magnesium	0.160
Zinc	0.019
Cadmium	ND
Copper	0.006
Chromium	ND
Nickel	1.097
Manganese	0.013
Iron	0.013

ND : Not detected

SCIENTIFIC NAME	:	*Dalbergia sissoo* Roxb
UNANI NAME	:	SHISHAM
FAMILY	:	*Papilionaceae*
PARTS USED	:	Bark, wood, leaves, and roots

PHARMACOLOGICAL PROPERTIES RELEVANT TO THERPEUTIC USE IN SKIN DIESEASES

Wood and bark possess alterative properties with claimed utility in eruptions, boils and leprosy while the roots are artringent. Decoction of leaves is useful in gonorrhoea[174]. The plant is used as a blood purifier for the treatment of various skin ailments including scabies in Indian systems of medicine[2,7,8,100,176]. Antimicrobial substances have been isolated from the plant[98]. Essential oils exhibited antifungal properties.[99] Other species of *Dalbergia* revealed anti-inflammatory effects[3].

ELEMENTAL COMPOSITION OF WOOD POWDER[176]

Element	Concentration (mg/g ash)
Magnesium	53.757
Calcium	751.445
Lead	0.202
Copper	0.156
Mercury	ND
Cobalt	ND
Zinc	0.491
Iron	0.095
Chromium	ND
Cadmium	Traces
Manganese	0.085
Nickel	ND
Silver	ND
Molybdenum	ND

ND : Not detected

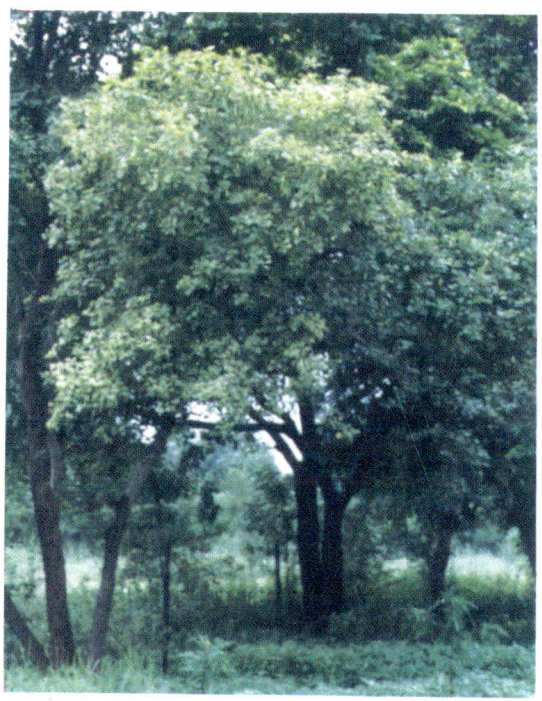

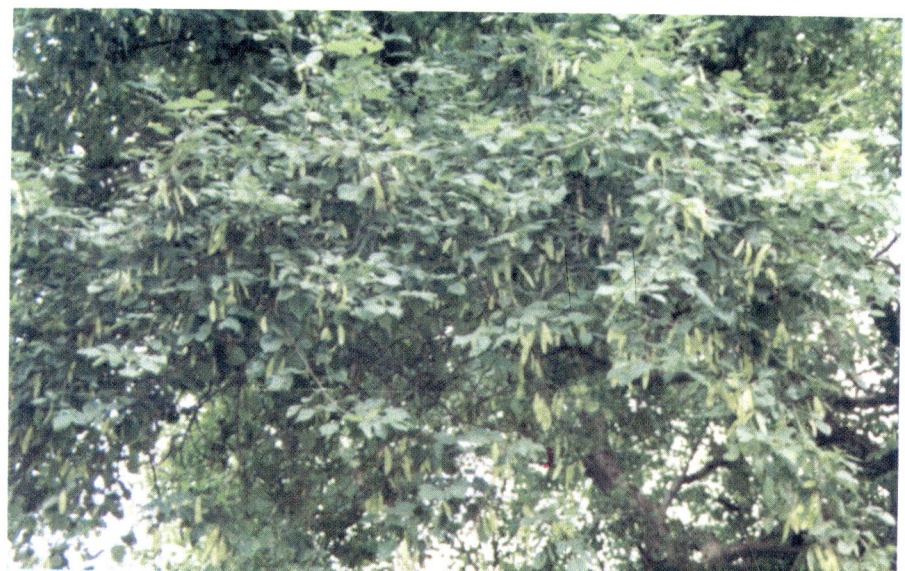

Dalbergia sissoo

(Field Photo : Dr. M.P. Sharma and Mr. Kaiser N. Khan)

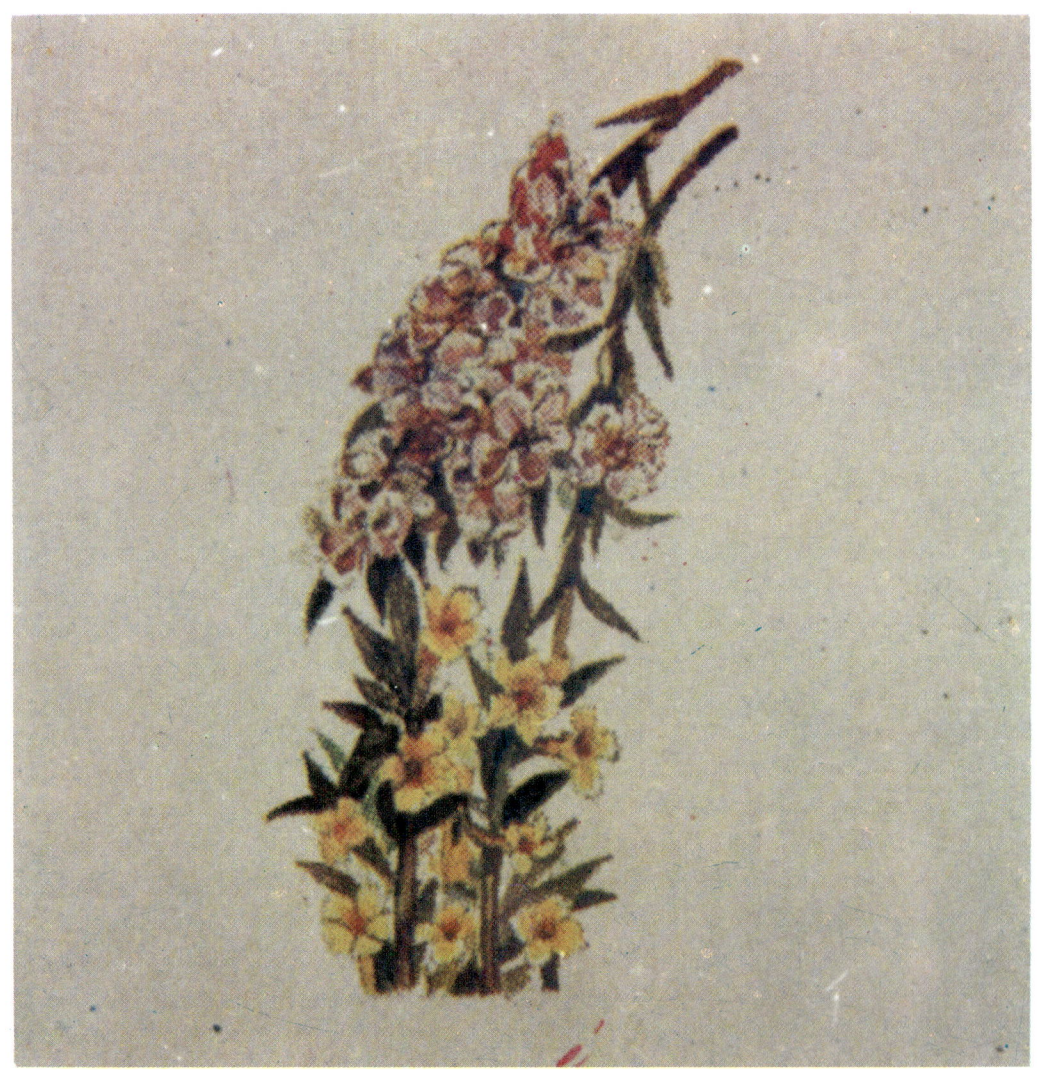

Daphne mezerium

(Field Photo : Hamdard Dawakhana, Delhi)

SCIENTIFIC NAME	:	*Daphne mezerium* Linn
		Daphne genkwa Sieb et Zucc
UNANI NAME	:	MAZRIUN
FAMILY	:	Thymoleaceae
PARTS USED	:	Whole plant

PHARMACOLOGICAL PROPERTIES RELEVANT TO THERAPEUTIC USE IN SKIN DISEASES

It is useful in cases of scabies and ulcers and is reported to contain some anti-cancer compounds.

ELEMENTAL COMPOSITION[228]

Element	Concentration (μg/g ash)
Copper	60.00
Zinc	500.00
Iron	7.40×10^3
Manganese	610.00
Magnesium	52.00×10^3
Nickel	12.40 ± 0.75
Cadmium	0.10
Cobalt	3.20
Lead	13.80
Silver	2.00
Molybdenum	5.60
Tin	ND
Chromium	21.20

ND - Not detected

SCIENTIFIC NAME	:	*Desmodium gangeticum* DC
UNANI NAME	:	SHALWAN
FAMILY	:	*Papilionaceae*
PARTS USED	:	Whole plant, root, bark

PHARMACOLOGICAL PROPERTIES RELEVANT TO THERAPEUTIC USE IN SKIN DISEASES

The root is attributed with alterative, tonic and febrifuge properties. Antibacterial, antifungal and anti-inflammatory effects were confirmed by experimental investigations using the aqueous extract[3,28]. Gangetin : a new pterocarpan isolated from the plant exhibited potent anti-inflammatory action against carrageenin induced edema and cotton pellet induced granuloma in rats184. It elicited marked reduction in the total proteins of the inflammatory exudate, inhibited degranulation effect induced by diazoxide, inhibited acid phosphatase activity in the granulation tissue and protected against erythrocyte lysis. Elevation of cyclic AMP level in the inflammatory tissue by inhibition of cAMP-phospho-diestrase activity was suggested as a possible mechanism of its antiinflammatory action[185].

ELEMENTAL COMPOSITION[228]

Element	Concentration (μg/g ash)
Copper	70.00
Zinc	460.00
Iron	8.20×10^3
Manganese	290.00
Magnesium	38.00×10^3
Chromium	32.40
Nickel	64.80
Cadmium	0.10
Lead	14.20
Silver	4.10
Molybdenum	2.50
Tin	0.04
Cobalt	7.80

ND - Not detected

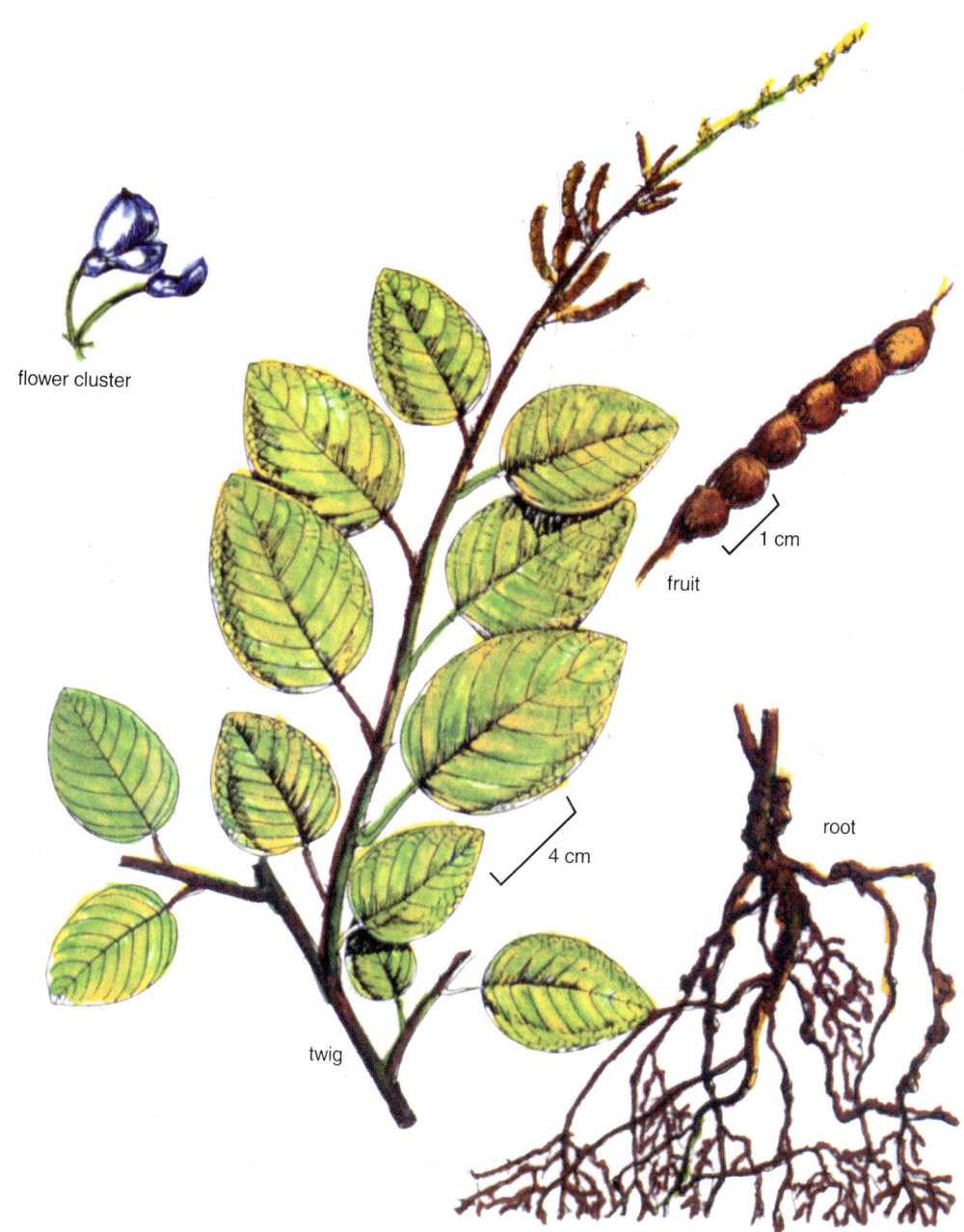

flower cluster

fruit

1 cm

root

4 cm

twig

Desmodium gangeticum
(Herbarium Photo : Dr. M.P. Sharma)

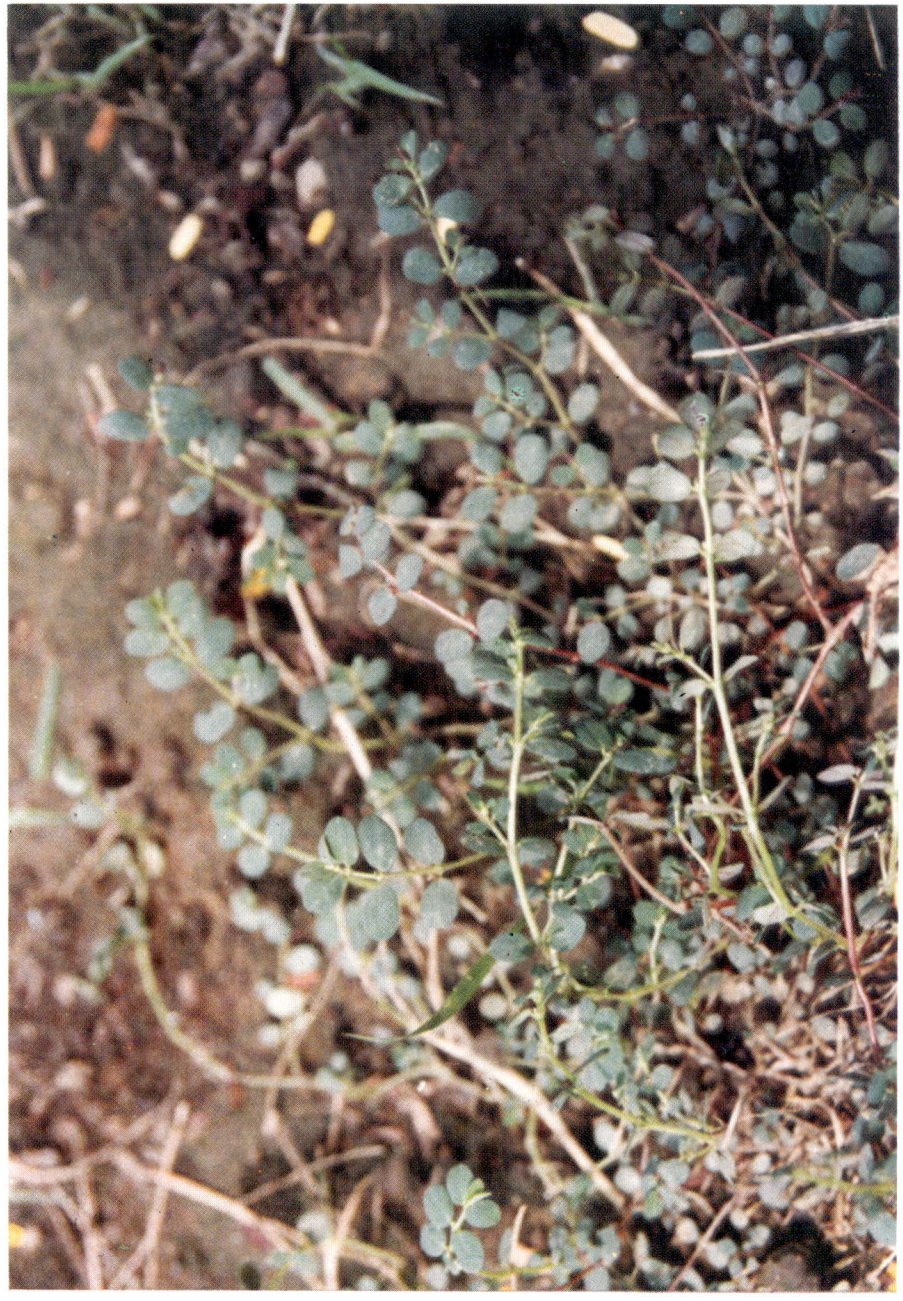

Euphorbia thymifolia

(Field Photo : Dr. M.P. Sharma and Mr. Kaiser N. Khan)

SCIENTIFIC NAME	:	*Euphorbia thymifolia* Linn
UNANI NAME	:	CHOTI DUDHI
FAMILY	:	*Euphorbiaceae*
PARTS USED	:	Whole plant

PHARMACOLOGICAL PROPERTIES RELEVANT TO THERAPEUTIC USE IN SKIN DISEASES

Juice of the plant is used in Indian systems of medicine for insect repellent action and for the treatment of various skin diseases including ring worm[174]. Ether extract of the plant has been reported to be very effective in treating sarcoptic mange in sheep[3]. Antifungal activity was confirmed by in vitro studies against *Trichophyton mentagrophytes, Trichophyton simii* and *Microsporum gypseum*[68,69].

ELEMENTAL COMPOSITION[228]

Element	Concentration (μg/g ash)
Copper	90.00
Zinc	350.00
Iron	2.90×10^3
Manganese	480.0
Magnesium	44.00×10^3
Chromium	0.86
Nickel	9.00
Cadmium	0.20
Cobalt	7.80
Lead	210.00
Silver	1.20
Molybdenum	4.40
Tin	0.04

ND - Not detected

SCIENTIFIC NAME	:	*Fumaria indica* (Haussk) Pugsley
Synonym	:	*F. parviflora* Lamk
UNANI NAME	:	SHAHTARA
FAMILY	:	*Fumeraceae*
PARTS USED	:	Whole plant

PHARMACOLOGICAL PROPERTIES RELEVANT TO THERAPEUTIC USE IN SKIN DISEASES

It is attributed with alterative, diaphoretic, choleretic and blood purifying properties and incorporated in formulations for use in skin diseases including leprosy, scrofula and syphilis[3,27,176]. Antibacterial and antiaging effects were reported in the plant principles obtained from *F. officinalis* and *F. vailanti*.[7,107]

ELEMENT COMPOSITION[176,228]

Element	Concentration (mg/g ash)
Magnesium	25.135
Calcium	59.459
Lead	0.081
Copper	0.067
Mercury	ND
Cobalt	ND
Zinc	0.412
Iron	0.254
Chromium	ND
Cadmium	ND
Manganese	0.143
Nickel	ND
Cobalt	0.006
Lead	0.012
Silver	0.0007
Molybdenum	0.012
Tin	ND

ND : Not detected

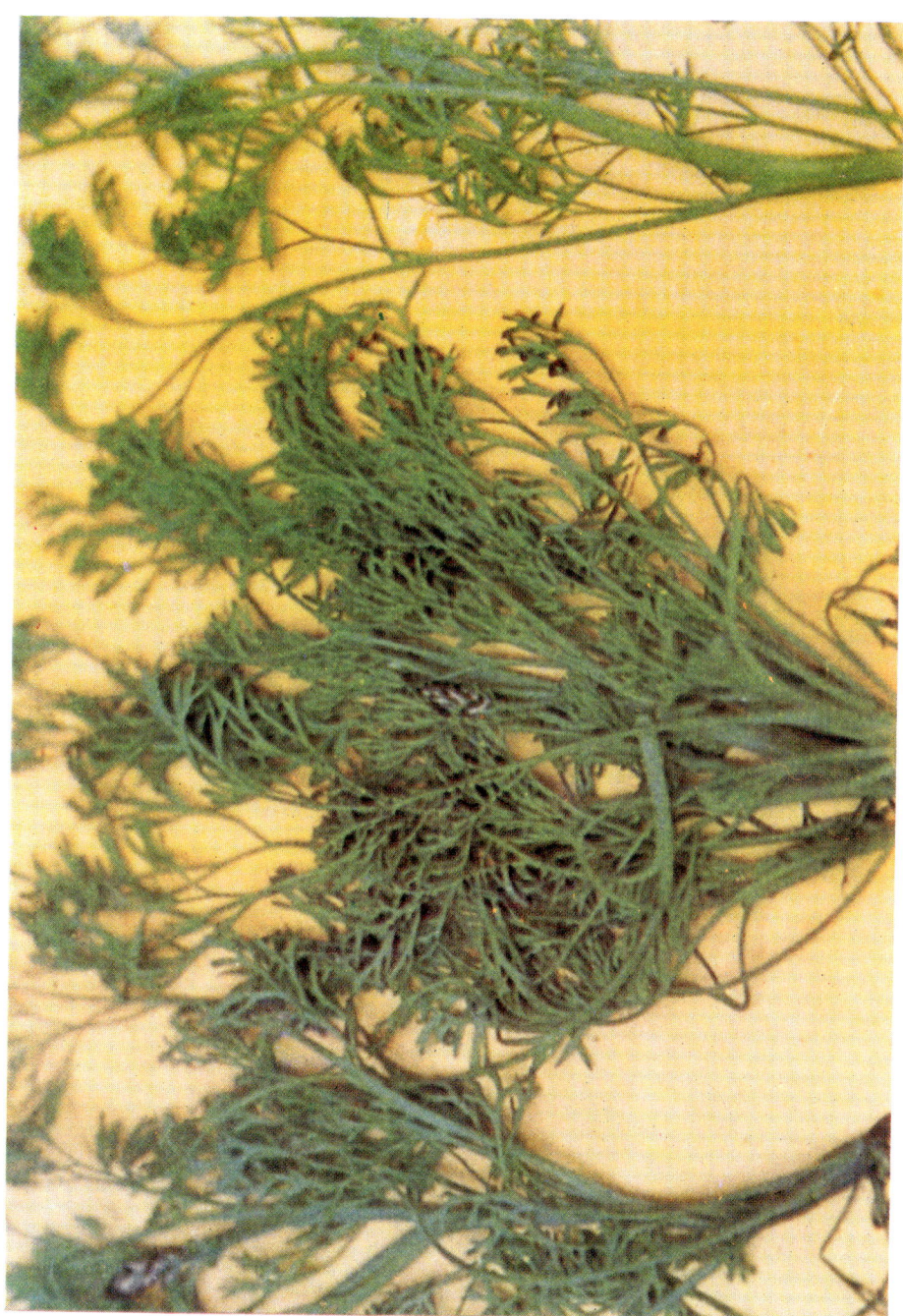

Fumaria indica
(Courtesy : C.C.R.U.M., New Delhi)

Inula racemosa

(Courtesy : C.C.R.U.M., New Delhi)

SCIENTIFIC NAME	:	*Inula racemosa* Hook f.
UNANI NAME	:	RASAN
FAMILY	:	*Asteraceae*
PARTS USED	:	Roots

PHARMACOLOGICAL PROPERTIES RELEVANT TO THERAPEUTIC USE IN SKIN DISEASES

The roots are claimed to be resolvent of indurations and of value in the treatment of skin diseases. Antiinflammatory activity was confirmed against carrageenin induced paw edema in rats. Potent antihistaminic and antiserotonergic activity was elicited by the crude extracts. Essential oils, olantolactone and isoolantolactone revealed antifungal effects against some dermatophytes *e.g. Trichophyton mentagrophytes, Microsporum canis, Fusarium solani, \Fusarium moniliforme, Helminthosporum oryzae, Helminthosporum turcium, Pythium vexans, Rhizoctonia bataticola, Rhizoctonia solani, Alternaria helianthi, Colletotrichum caprici, Pyricularia setariae* etc. Some improvement was also observed in experimental ring worm infection in guinea pigs following treatment with a mixture of these principles. The essential oils exhibited antibacterial effects against many gram positive and gram negative organisms *e.g. Staphylococcus albus, Staphylococcus aureus, Escherichia coli, Klebsiella pneumoniae, Pseudomonas aeruginosa. Proteus vulgaris, Bacillus anthracis, Bacillus subtilis* and *Corynebacterum pyogenes*[14,186-188].

ELEMENTAL COMPOSITION[227, 228]

Element	Concentration (mg/g ash)
Copper	0.208
Zinc	0.019
Iron	0.310
Manganese	0.153
Magnesium	2.100
Chromium	0.015
Nickel	0.029
Cadmium	0.001
Cobalt	0.004
Lead	0.001
Silver	0.002
Molybdenum	0.001
Tin	0.0001

SCIENTIFIC NAME	:	*Lawsonia alba* Lam
Synonym	:	*Lawsonia innermis* Linn
UNANI NAME	:	MEHNDI
FAMILY	:	*Lythraceae*
PARTS USED	:	Leaves

PHARMACOLOGICAL PROPERTIES RELEVANT TO THERAPEUTIC USE IN SKIN DISEASES

The leaves are attributed with alterative, demulcent and blood purifying properties and are used traditionally for treating and preventing skin diseases and for cosmetic purposes including ornamental colouring of palms and soles and also as a hair dye and hair conditioner[7,8]. Freshly extracted juice of leaves is incorporated in a Siddha oily-formulation used for the treatment of *Alopecia aerata*. Application of this oil is claimed to prevent falling of hair and promote the growth of new hair[2]. Antibacterial and antifungal properties were demonstrated against a variety of microorganisms by *in vitro* and *in vivo* studies. The antifungal effects elicited by the purified principle *Lawsone* were found to be particularly potent and were shown to be due to an inhibitory action on peroxidase and nitrate reductase enzymes. The ethanolic extract of leaves exhibited significant antiinflammatory and anti-hyaluronidase actions[186].

ELEMENTAL COMPOSITION[227, 228]

Element	Concentration (mg/g ash)
Copper	0.157
Zinc	0.126
Iron	9.400
Manganese	1.045
Magnesium	48.000
Chromium	0.028
Nickel	0.032
Cadmium	0.0008
Cobalt	0.008
Lead	0.015
Silver	0.007
Molybdenum	0.020
Tin	0.0001

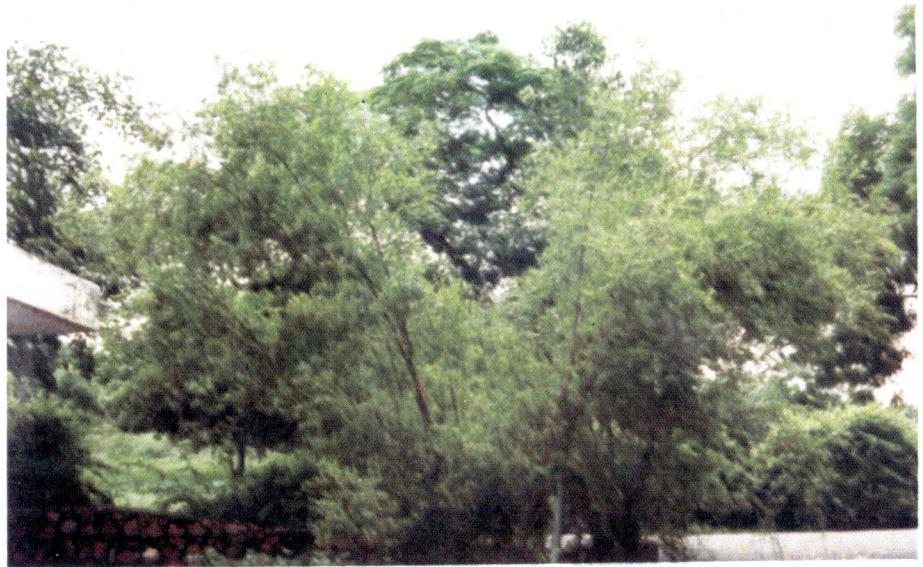

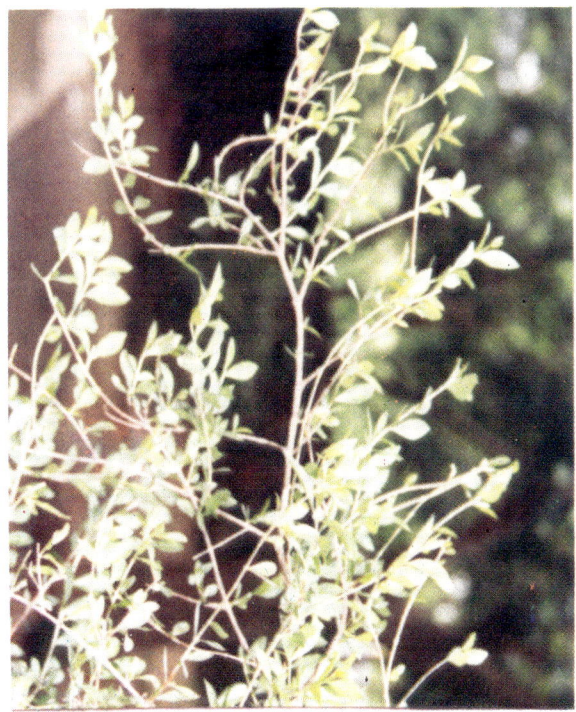

Lawsonia alba

(Field Photo : Dr. M.P. Sharma and Mr. Kaiser N. Khan)

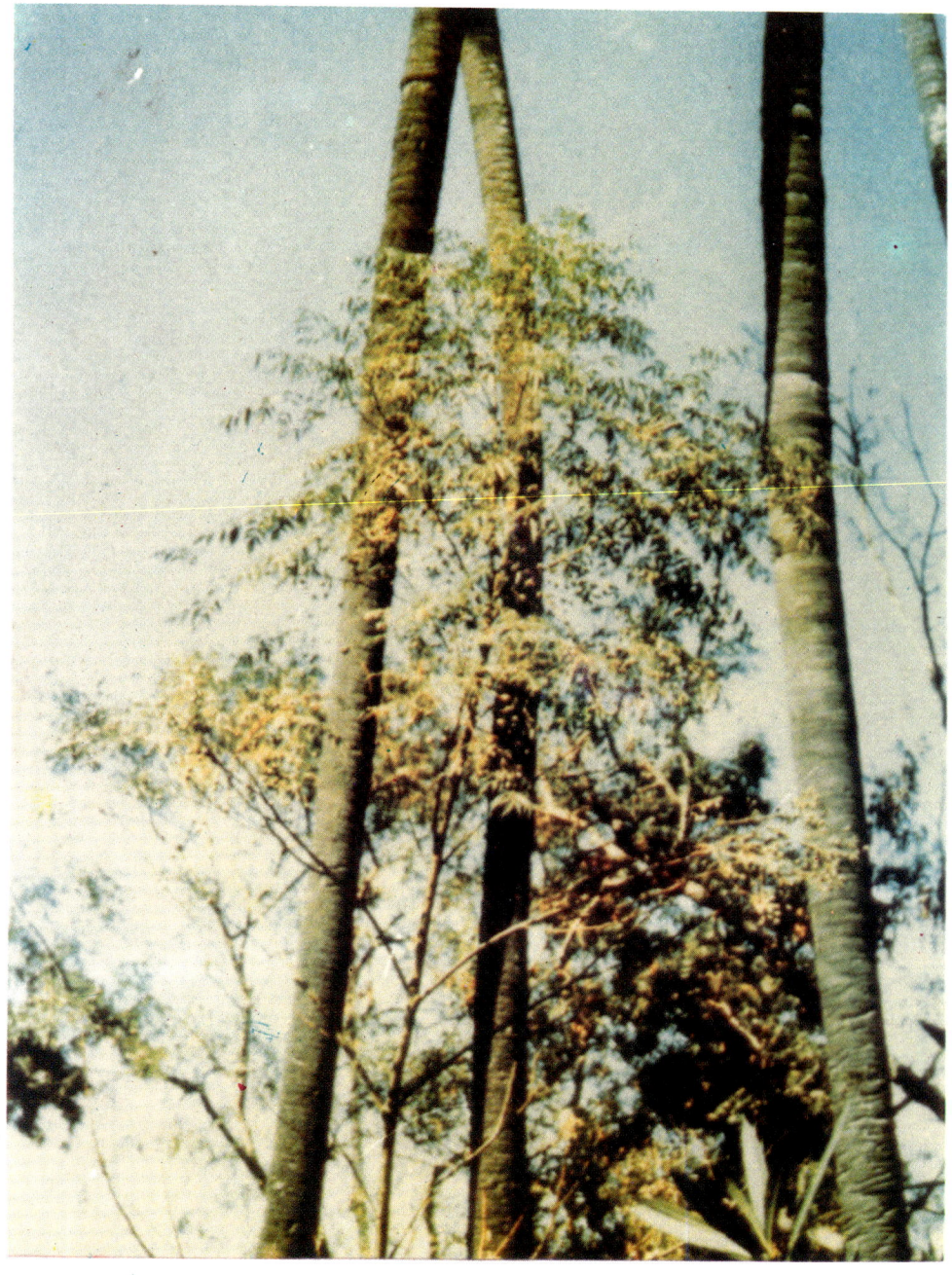

Melia azadarach

(Courtesy : C.C.R.U.M., New Delhi)

SCIENTIFIC NAME	:	*Melia azedarach* Linn
UNANI NAME	:	BAKAYAN
FAMILY	:	*Meliaceae*
PARTS USED	:	Leaves, bark, flowers, fruits

PHARMACOLOGICAL PROPERTIES RELEVANT TO THERAPEUTIC USE IN SKIN DISEASES

The plant is reputed for its emolient, astringent, antiseptic, counterirritant, resolvent, deodourant and healing properties and is considered to be of value for the treatment of eruptive skin diseases, scrofula, leprosy and for killing of lice[2,7,8,174,186]. Oil is used for the dressing of ulcers and applied for beneficial effects in cases of urticaria, eczema, ringworm, scabies, pemphigus, scrofula and leprosy. Antibacterial, antiviral, insecticidal, anthelmintic, anticancer and mild analgesic effects were confirmed by experimental investigations[27,186].

ELEMENTAL COMPOSITION[227]

Element	Concentration (mg/g ash)
Copper	0.204
Zinc	0.038
Iron	7.950
Manganese	0.416
Magnesium	42.600
Chromium	0.035
Nickel	0.020
Cadmium	0.0006
Cobalt	0.011
Lead	0.002
Silver	0.002
Molybdenum	0.002
Tin	0.0001

SCIENTIFIC NAME	:	*Moringa oleifera* Lam
Synonym	:	*Moringa pterigosperma* Gaertin
UNANI NAME	:	SONJANA
FAMILY	:	*Moringaceace*
PARTS USED	:	Roots, seeds, leaves, stem bark

PHARMACOLOGICAL PROPERTIES RELEVANT TO THERAPEUTIC USE IN SKIN DISEASES

Roots, leaves, and seeds are attributed with rubefascient, antirheumatic, and antiinflammatory properties and considered useful in burns, sores, rheumatism, erysepelas, scabies and cases of snake bite and scorpion sting[186]. Antibacterial, antifungal and antiviral properties were confirmed by experimental investigations using crude extracts obtained from different parts of the plant. Pterigospermin and benzyl-iso thiocyanate, isolated from the roots, were reported as the antibiotic principles acting possibly through inhibition of transaminases[41,130-132,186]. Ethanolic extract was also shown to elicit anti-inflammatory effects against formalin induced paw oedema and cotton pellet induced granuloma in rat[28]. The leaves are rich in Vitamin C content (220 mg/100g)[25]. Aerial parts of the plant are reported to elicit anticancer effects[21].

ELEMENTAL COMPOSITION[227, 228]

Element	Concentration (mg/g ash)
Copper	0.217
Zinc	0.258
Iron	8.900
Manganese	2.180
Magnesium	36.600
Chromium	0.037
Nickel	0.028
Cadmium	0.004
Cobalt	0.003
Lead	0.001
Silver	0.003
Molybdenum	ND
Tin	0.0001

ND : Not detected

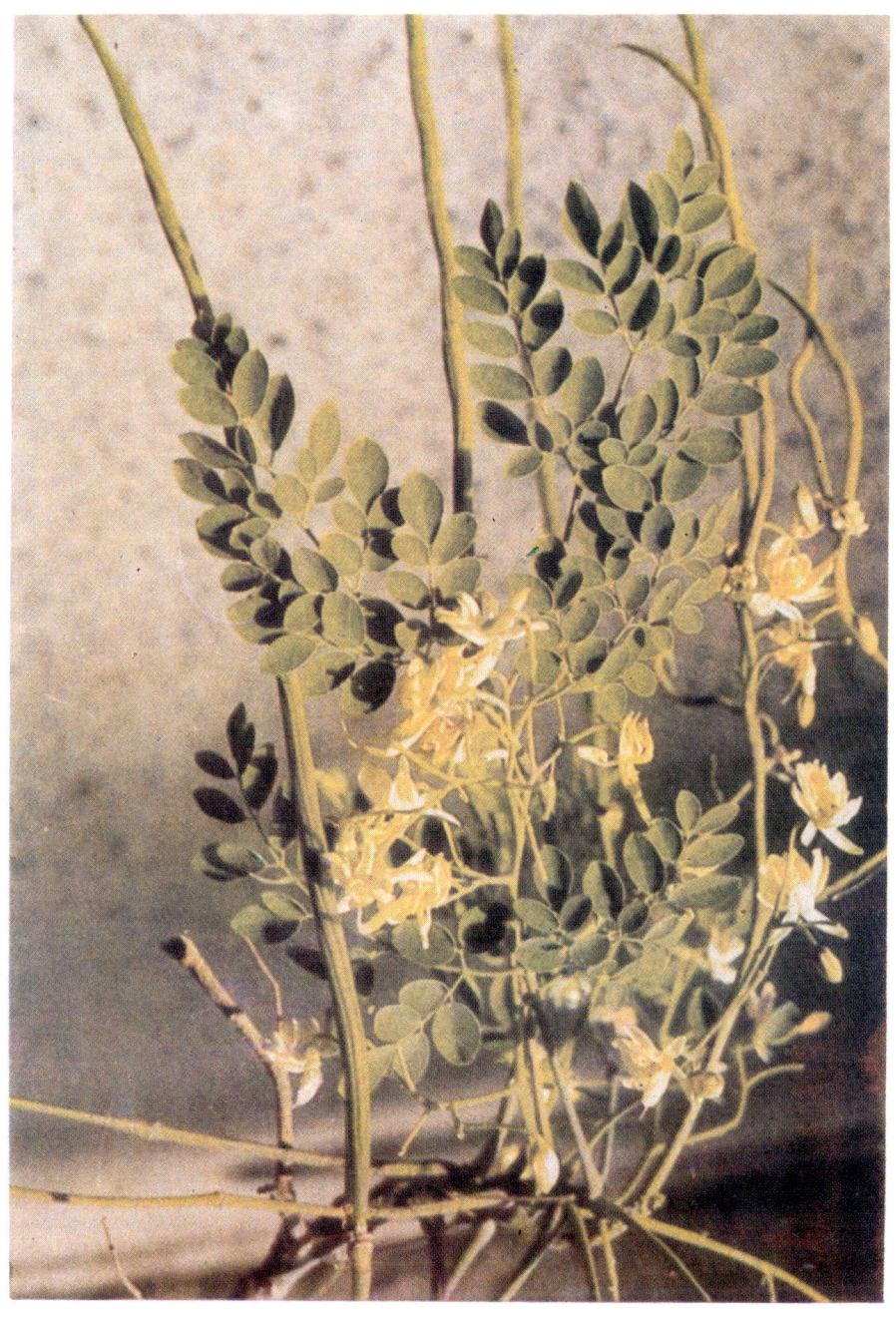

Moringa oleifera
(Courtesy : ICMR, New Delhi)

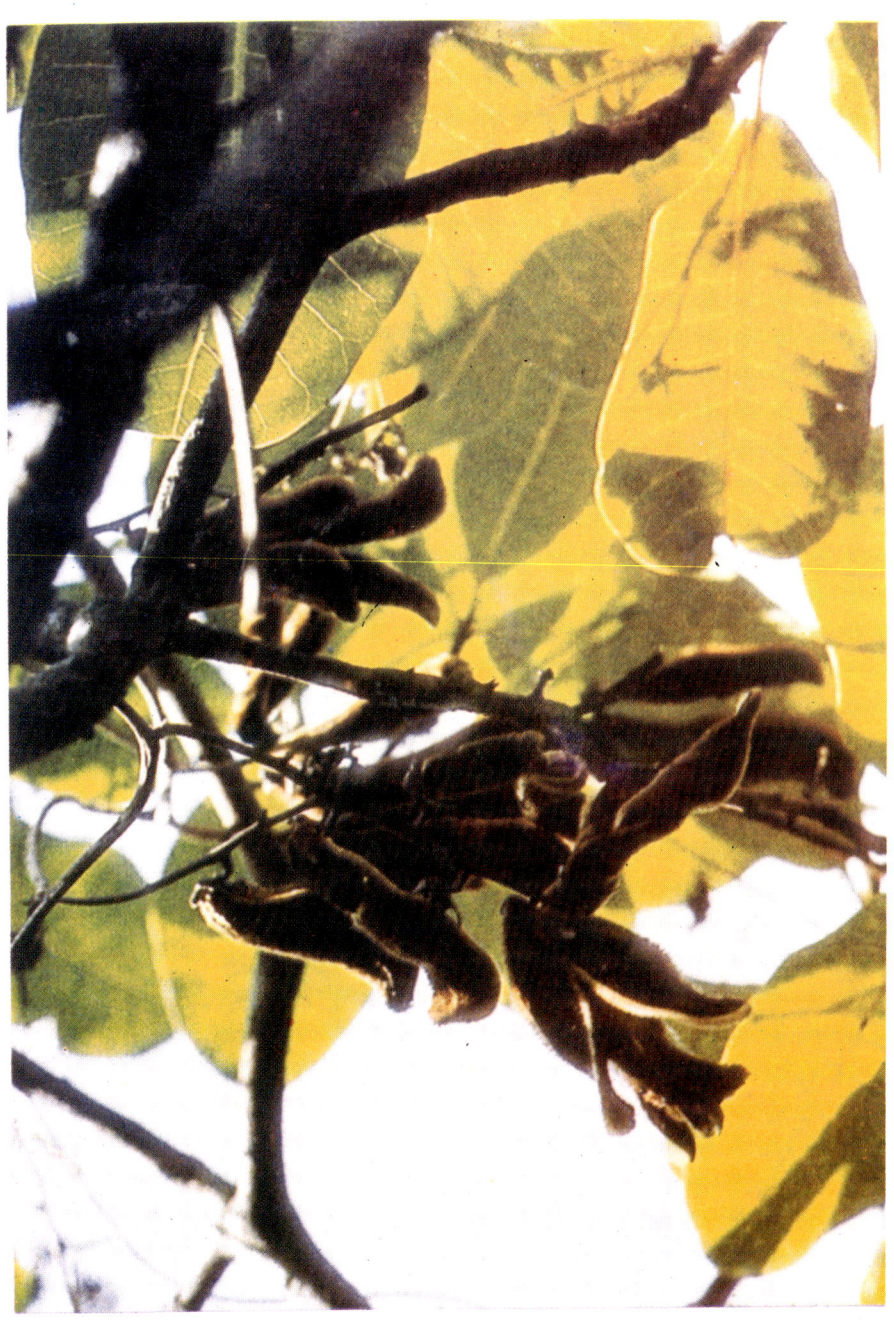

Mucuna pruriens
(Courtesy : ICMR, New Delhi)

SCIENTIFIC NAME	:	*Mucuna pruriens* DC
UNANI NAME	:	KONCH
FAMILY	:	*Papilionaceae*
PARTS USED	:	Seeds, roots, leaves, and fruits

PHARMACOLOGICAL PROPERTIES RELEVANT TO THERAPEUTIC USE IN SKIN DISEASES

The plant is attributed with blood purifying and astringent properties. Application of paste of roots on the body is claimed to elicit beneficial effect in cases of dropsy. Various parts of the plant are used in traditional medicine for the treatment of ulcers, sores, ringworm, snakebite, scorpion sting and for promotion of fracture healing[7,27,186]. Antifungal activity was confirmed by experimental investigations. It is incorporated in several multi-herbal and herbo-mineral preparations with claimed adaptogenic and antiaging effects. The plant is also known to produce itching and histaminergic actions which may adversely affect a skin ailment[14,186].

ELEMENTAL COMPOSITION[227, 228]

Element	Concentration (mg/g ash)
Copper	0.177
Zinc	0.218
Iron	5.270
Manganese	0.209
Magnesium	33.300
Chromium	ND
Nickel	0.107
Cadmium	0.0005
Cobalt	0.012
Lead	0.002
Silver	0.003
Molybdenum	0.003
Tin	0.0001

ND : Not detected

SCIENTIFIC NAME	:	*Nymphaea alba* Linn
UNANI NAME	:	NILOFAR
FAMILY	:	*Nymphaceae*
PARTS USED	:	Flowers and leaves

PHARMACOLOGICAL PROPERTIES RELEVANT TO THERAPEUTIC USE IN SKIN DISEASES

Flowers, leaves and filaments are attributed with blood purifying, refrigerant and astringent properties and are claimed to give relief in erysepelas and burning of soles[7,186]. *In vitro* antibacterial activity was reported in the ethanolic and aqueous extract of flowers against gram positive organisms[5]. Another species *N. stellata* exhibited potent anti-inflammatory action against carrageenin induced paw edema in rats. The effect compared well with that elicited by hydrocortisone. Crude extracts of *N. stellata* were, however, found to be devoid of antibacterial, antifungal and antiviral actions[186]. Fruit nodules and foliage are reported to contain 235 and 170 mg% Vitamin C respectively[25].

ELEMENTAL COMPOSITION[229]

Element	Concentration (mg/g ash)
Magnesium	32.456
Zinc	0.746
Iron	0.702
Calcium	10.351
Lead	0.263
Manganese	0.897
Copper	0.247
Nickel	0.289
Cobalt	ND
Mercury	Traces
Silver	ND
Strontium	ND
Tin	Traces
Molybdenum	ND

ND : Not detected

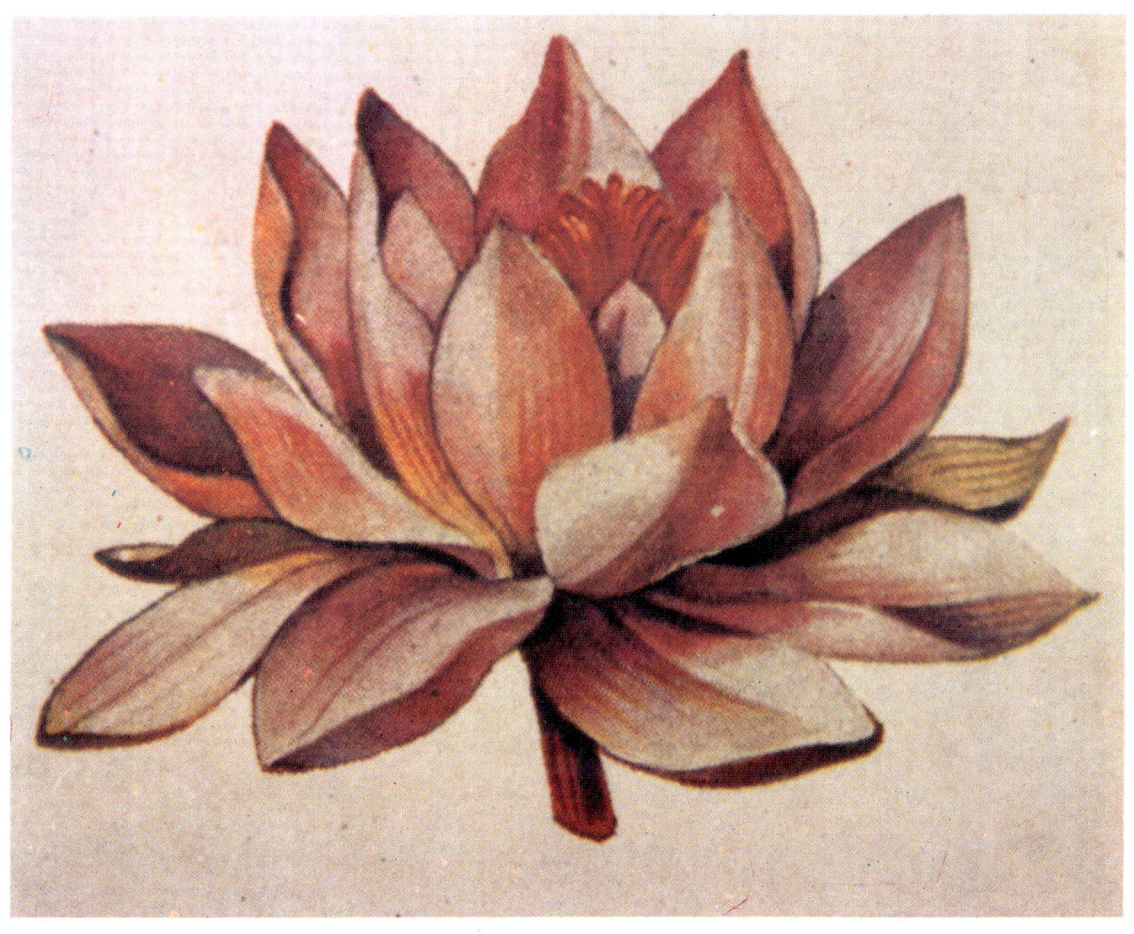

Nymphaea alba
(Courtesy : Hamdard Dawakhana, Delhi)

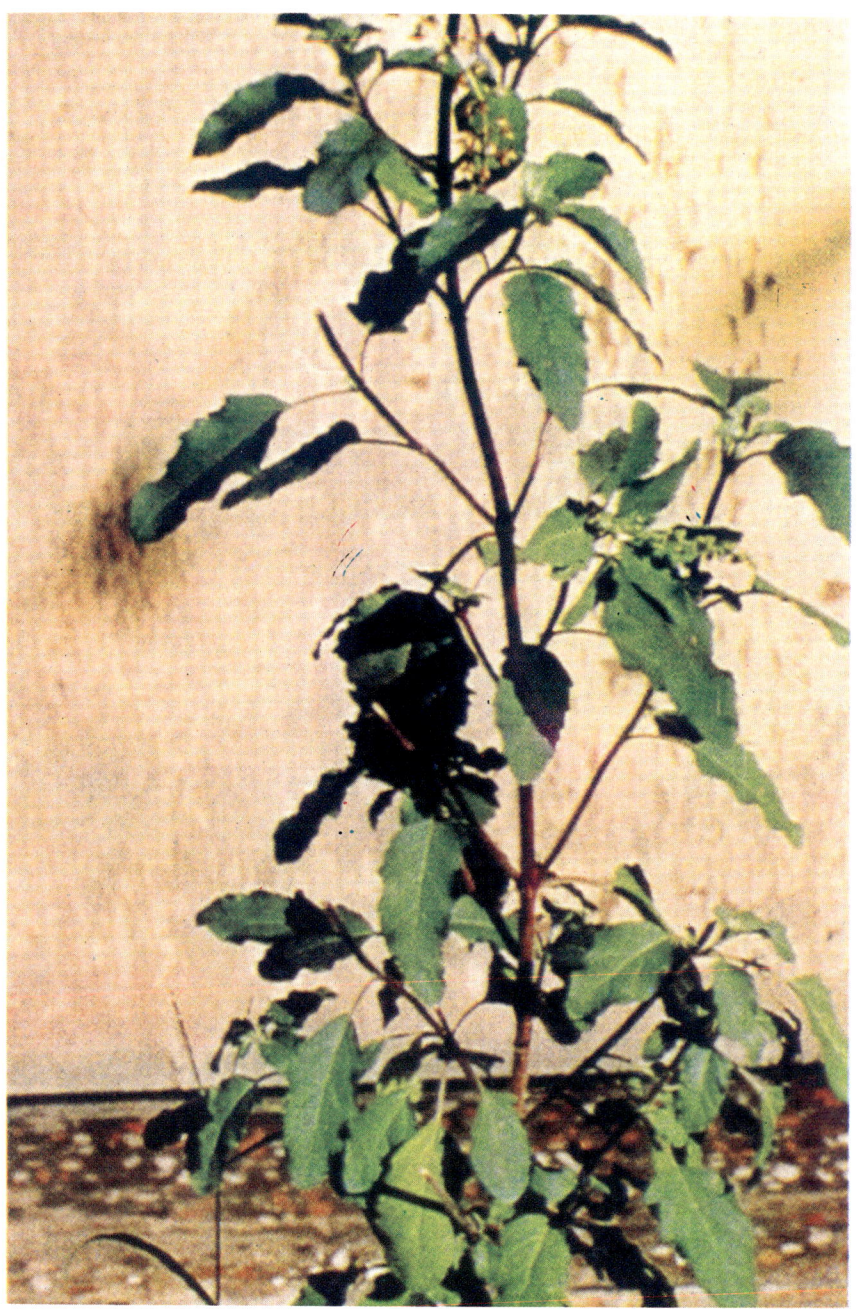

Ocimum sanctum

(Courtesy : ICMR, New Delhi)

SCIENTIFIC NAME	:	*Ocimum sanctum* Linn
UNANI NAME	:	TULSI
FAMILY	:	*Labiatae*
PARTS USED	:	Leaves, seeds

PHARMACOLOGICAL PROPERTIES RELEVANT TO THERAPEUTIC USE IN SKIN DISEASES

The plant is attributed with blood purifying, demulcent, antiseptic, diaphoretic and tonic/rejuvenating properties with claimed utility in itches, ring worm, leprosy and other skin diseases[7,8,27,174,186]. Antibacterial, antifungal, antiviral, anti-ulcer, anti-stress and adaptogenic effects of the plant were confirmed by scientific investigations. Antimicrobial effects were reported in the crude extracts (aqueous, ethanolic and petroleum ether), essential oil and eugenol. This was shown both by *in vitro* and *in vivo* studies. The seeds elicited anti-coagulase activity and suppressed mannitol fermentability of pathogenic *Staphylococci*. Antibacterial actions were elicited against both gram positive and gram negative bacterial including effects on *Mycobacterium tuberculosis*[10,27,118,135,138,186,189-193]. Antifungal activity was demonstrated on all major dermatophytes including *Aspergillus niger Candida guillermondii, Candila torulopsis, Colletetrichum caprici, Curyularia* sp. *Epidermophyton floccosum, Fusarium oxysporum, Fusarium solani, Helminthosporum oryzae, Microsporum canis, Penicillum digitatum, Rhizopus nigricans, Rhizopus stolonifer, Sacchromyces cerevisae, Trichophyton mentagrophytes* etc. with maximum efficacy shown by eugenol[127,186,194,195]. Antiviral effects were reported with the crude extracts, leaf juice and the essential oil. Antiviral component was concentrated in the young leaves[186]. Various extracts and the oil exhibited insecticidal, nematicidal and larvicidal actions also[196-200].

The plant is reported to possess antihistaminic, ulcer protecting, adaptogenic, antistress, growth promoting, and immuno-modulating properties[54,201-204]. Leaves contain 83 mg% ascorbic acid[25]. Clinical studies revealed beneficial effects in acne vulgaris[205], viral encephalitis[206], peptic ulcers[207], and in healing of infected wounds[128].

ELEMENTAL COMPOSITION[229]

Element	Concentration (mg/g ash)
Magnesium	82.222
Zinc	0.629
Iron	0.463
Calcium	206.018
Manganese	0.926
Copper	0.616
Nickel	0.213
Cobalt	ND
Mercury	Traces
Silver	ND
Strontium	Traces
Tin	Traces
Molybdenum	ND

ND : Not detected

SCIENTIFIC NAME	:	*Plumbago rosea* Linn
Synonym	:	*Plumbago indica* Linn
UNANI NAME	:	LAL CHITRA
FAMILY	:	*Plumbaginaceae*
PARTS USED	:	Roots

PHARMACOLOGICAL PROPERTIES RELEVANT TO THERAPEUTIC USE IN SKIN DISEASES

The root is attributed with acrid, stimulating and counter irritant properties and is used in combination with some bland oil for local application in rheumatic/inflammatory conditions. Plumbagin from allied species *Plumbago zeylanica* (considered to be a cultivated variety of *P. rosea*) is reported to elicit beneficial effect in leucoderma[174], leprotic lesions, and other skin diseases[7,27,186]. While the latex is useful for topical application in cases of scabies and ulcers[156]. Antibacterial and antifungal effects were confirmed by experimental studies but the extracts or plumbagin were found to be devoid of anticancer activities. Antimicrobial effects were reported in chloroform extract and plumbagin against both gram positive and gram negative organisms but the 50% ethanolic extract did not elicit such effects. Antifungal activity was observed against a variety of dermatophytes including *Trichophyton, Epidermopyton* and *Microsporum* sp. at very low concentrations[186]. The plant extracts are reported to elicit antihistaminic actions[208]. Topical application of plumbagin was found to be clinically useful in cases of common warts[209].

ELEMENTAL COMPOSITION[210]

Element	Concentration (mg/g ash)
Sodium	0.027
Magnesium	0.055
Aluminum	0.012
Potassium	0.188
Calcium	0.510
Vanadium	ND
Chromium	0.002
Manganese	0.001
Iron	0.007
Cobalt	0.0002
Nickel	0.0003
Copper	ND
Zinc	0.0001
Molybdenum	ND
Silver	0.003

ND : Not detected

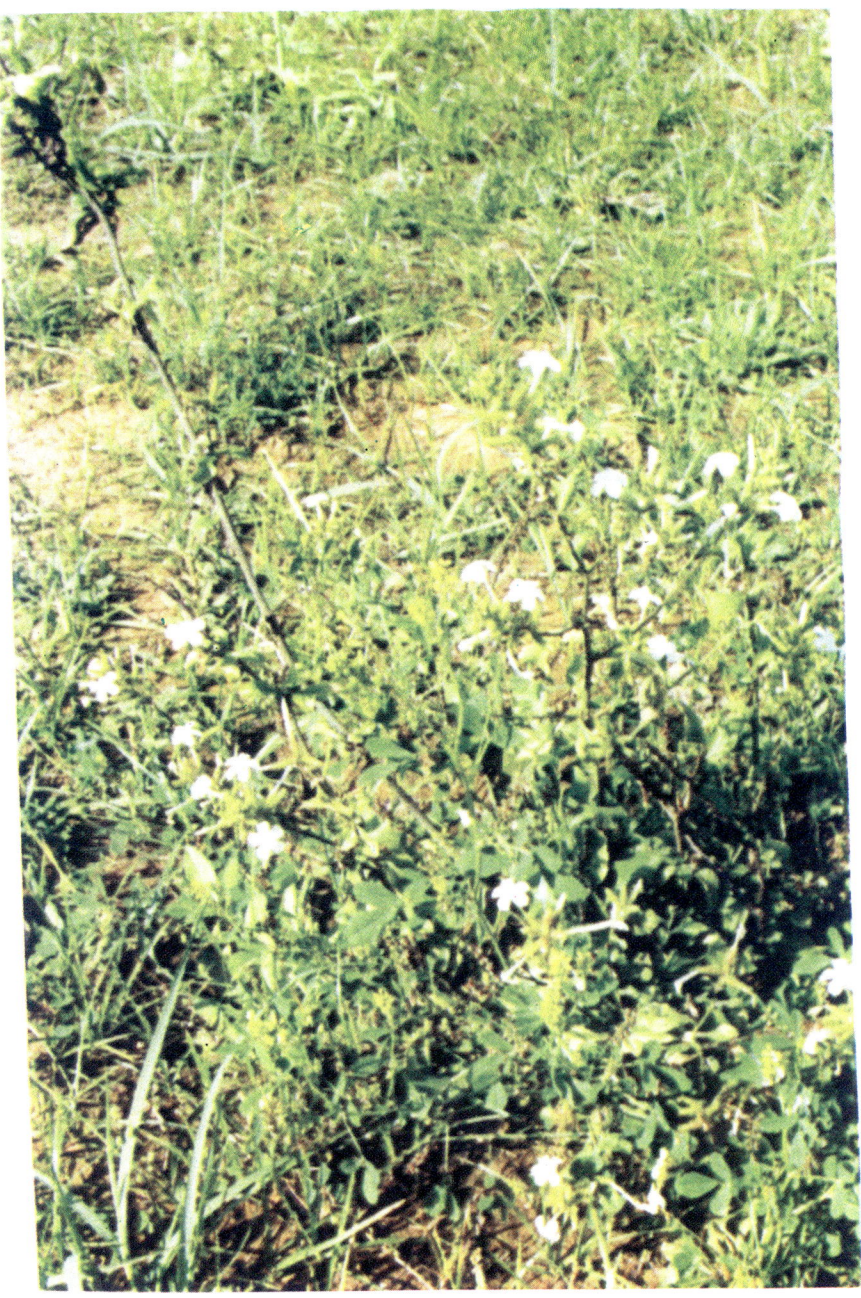

Plumbago rosea
(Field Photo : Dr. S.K. Raisuddin)

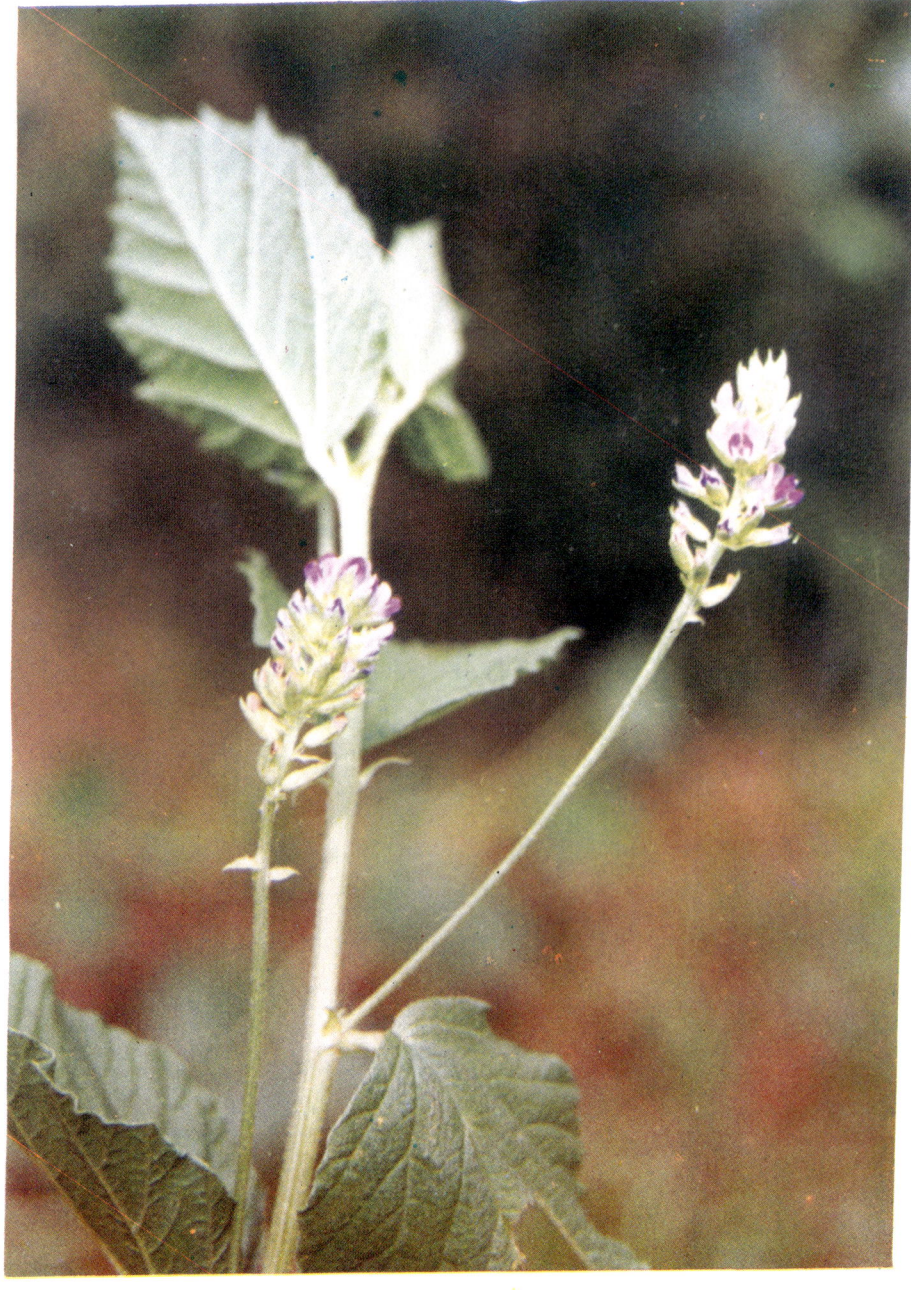

Psoralea corylifolia
(Field Photo : Dr. M.P. Sharma and Mr. Kaiser N. Khan)

SCIENTIFIC NAME	:	*Psoralea corylifolia* Linn
UNANI NAME	:	BABCHI
FAMILY	:	*Papilionaceae*
PARTS USED	:	Leaves, and seeds

PHARMACOLOGICAL PROPERTIES RELEVANT TO THERAPEUTIC USE IN SKIN DISEASES

The plant extracts/principles are used both internally and by topical application in the form of paste or ointment for the treatment of various skin diseases including leprosy and leucoderma. Antibacterial and antifungal effects were confirmed by experimental investigations carried out *in vitro* and *in vivo* using crude extracts and the essential oil. The active substances psoralen, isopsoralen and bavachinine were extensively studied for beneficial effects in leucoderma with very good results obtained in experimental animals and clinical trials. Antiinflammatory effects were confirmed in the flavonoidal principle: bavachinine[2,7,8,28,174,186]. The details are given in Chapter 6 (please see section 6.4.2).

ELEMENTAL COMPOSITION[228]

Element	Concentration (mg/g ash)
Copper	0.179
Zinc	0.231
Iron	6.820
Manganese	1.544
Magnesium	65.000
Chromium	0.035
Nickel	0.036
Cadmium	ND
Cobalt	0.008
Lead	0.350
Silver	0.008
Molybdenum	0.097
Tin	0.0001

ND : Not detected

SCIENTIFIC NAME	:	*Pterocarpus santalinus* Linn
UNANI NAME	:	SANDAL SURKH
FAMILY	:	*Papilionaceae*
PARTS USED	:	Wood

PHARMACOLOGICAL PROPERTIES RELEVANT TO THERAPEUTIC USE IN SKIN DISEASES

The plant is attributed with astringent, antiseptic, blood purifying and antiinflammatory properties with claimed utility in skin diseases, swellings, piles, snake bite and scorpion sting[1,8,27,174]. In a screening programme at CDRI, Lucknow, crude extracts from different parts of the plant were found to be devoid of antibacterial, antifungal and antiviral effects. The ethanol extract revealed tranquilosedative action. An ointment prepared from the ethanolic extract of the wood of another species *P. marsupium* showed clinical efficacy against dermophyte infections. (*Tinea cruris, Tinea corporis* and mixed infections) following local application for 7 to 10 days[1,186].

ELEMENTAL COMPOSITION OF WOOD POWDER[176]

Element	Concentration (mg/g ash)
Magnesium	36.207
Calcium	907.441
Lead	0.376
Copper	0.172
Mercury	0.136
Cobalt	ND
Zinc	0.987
Iron	0.256
Chromium	ND
Cadmium	Traces
Manganese	0.068
Nickel	ND
Silver	ND
Molybdenum	ND

ND : Not detected

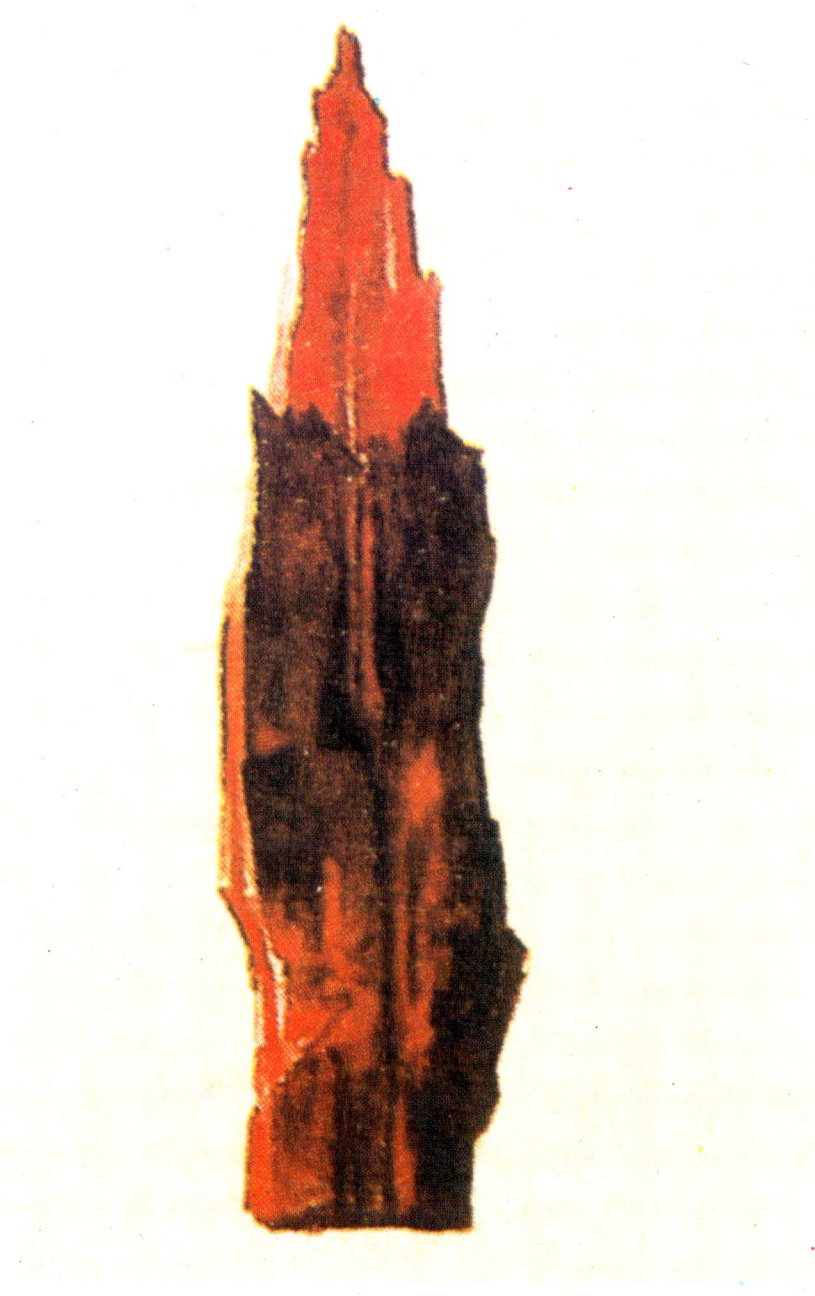

Pterocarpus santalinus

(Courtesy : Hamdard Dawakhana, Delhi)

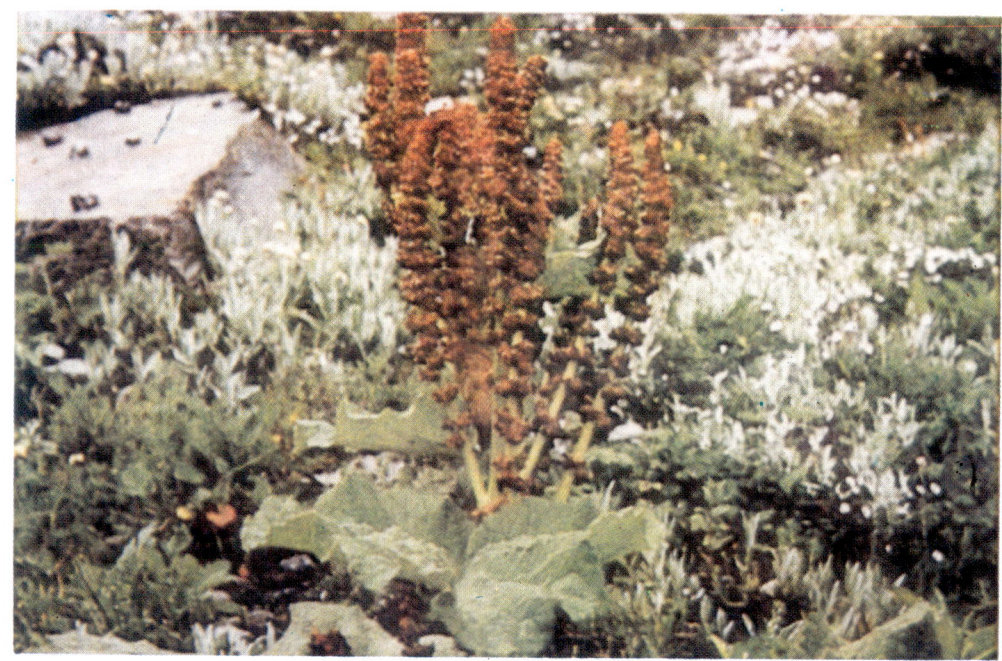

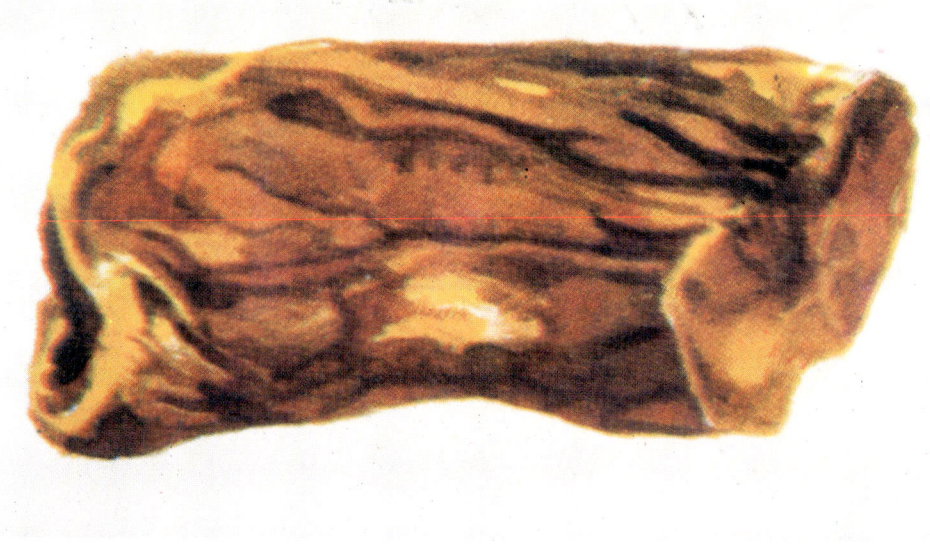

Rheum emodi

(*Upper* : Field Photo : Dr. M.P. Sharma and Mr. Kaiser N. Khan;
Lower : Courtesy : Hamdard Dawakhana, Delhi)

SCIENTIFIC NAME	:	*Rheum emodi* Wall
UNANI NAME	:	REVAND CHINI
FAMILY	:	*Polygonaceae*
PARTS USED	:	Root

PHARMACOLOGICAL PROPERTIES RELEVANT TO THERAPEUTIC USE IN SKIN DISEASES

Rhubarb is a pharmacopoeial drug used in modern medicine as a purgative. In traditional medicine it is attributed with astringent and tonic properties and is claimed to be useful in bruises, painful inflammatory conditions and piles[8,27,174,176] Scientific reports to confirm or refute these claims are not available.

ELEMENTAL COMPOSITION[176]

Element	Concentration (mg/g ash)
Magnesium	74.307
Calcium	469.405
Lead	0.168
Copper	0.034
Mercury	ND
Cobalt	ND
Zinc	0.712
Iron	0.105
Chromium	ND
Cadmium	ND
Manganese	0.441
Nickel	ND
Silver	ND
Molybdenum	ND

ND : Not detected

SCIENTIFIC NAME	:	*Rosa damascena* Mill
UNANI NAME	:	GUL-I-SURKH
FAMILY	:	*Rosaceae*
PARTS USED	:	Flowers

PHARMACOLOGICAL PROPERTIES RELEVANT TO THERAPEUTIC USE IN SKIN DISEASES

Rose water, distillate and oil from rose petals are incorporated in lotions collyria, and perfumes. It is an ingredient of a popular blood purifying formulation used in India for treating acne, pimples and for improving complexion[1,7,8,176]. Antibacterial and antifungal effects were confirmed by experimental investigations. The antimicrobial activity resides in the essential oil[9,211].

ELEMENTAL COMPOSITION OF FLOWERS[176, 228]

Element	Concentration (mg/g ash)
Magnesium	27.939
Calcium	21.316
Lead	0.413
Copper	0.070
Mercury	ND
Cobalt	0.006
Zinc	0.507
Iron	0.215
Chromium	ND
Cadmium	ND
Manganese	0.228
Nickel	ND
Silver	0.001
Molybdenum	0.011
Tin	0.0002

ND : Not detected

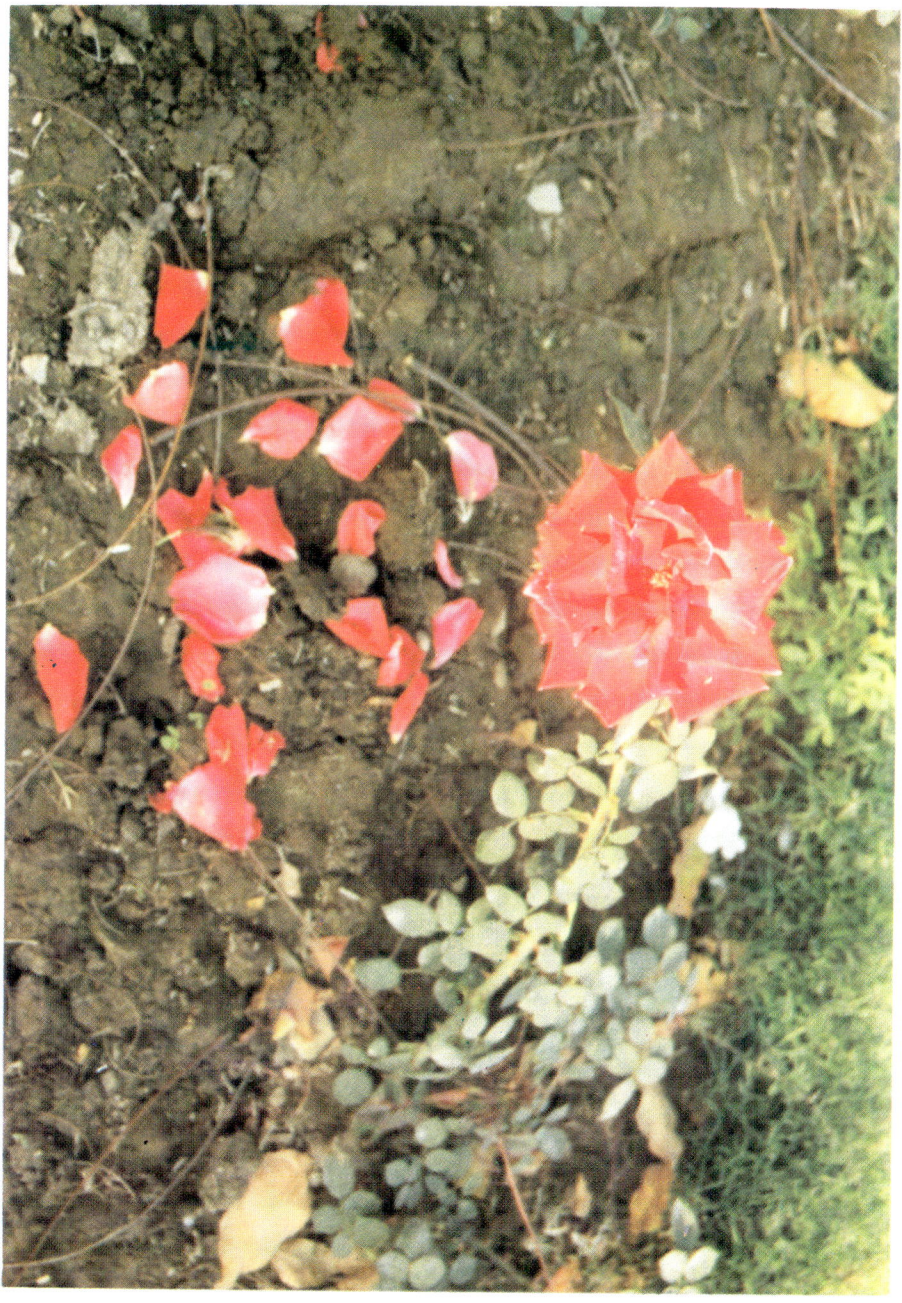

Rosa damascena

(Field Photo : Dr. M.P. Sharma and Mr. Kaiser N. Khan)

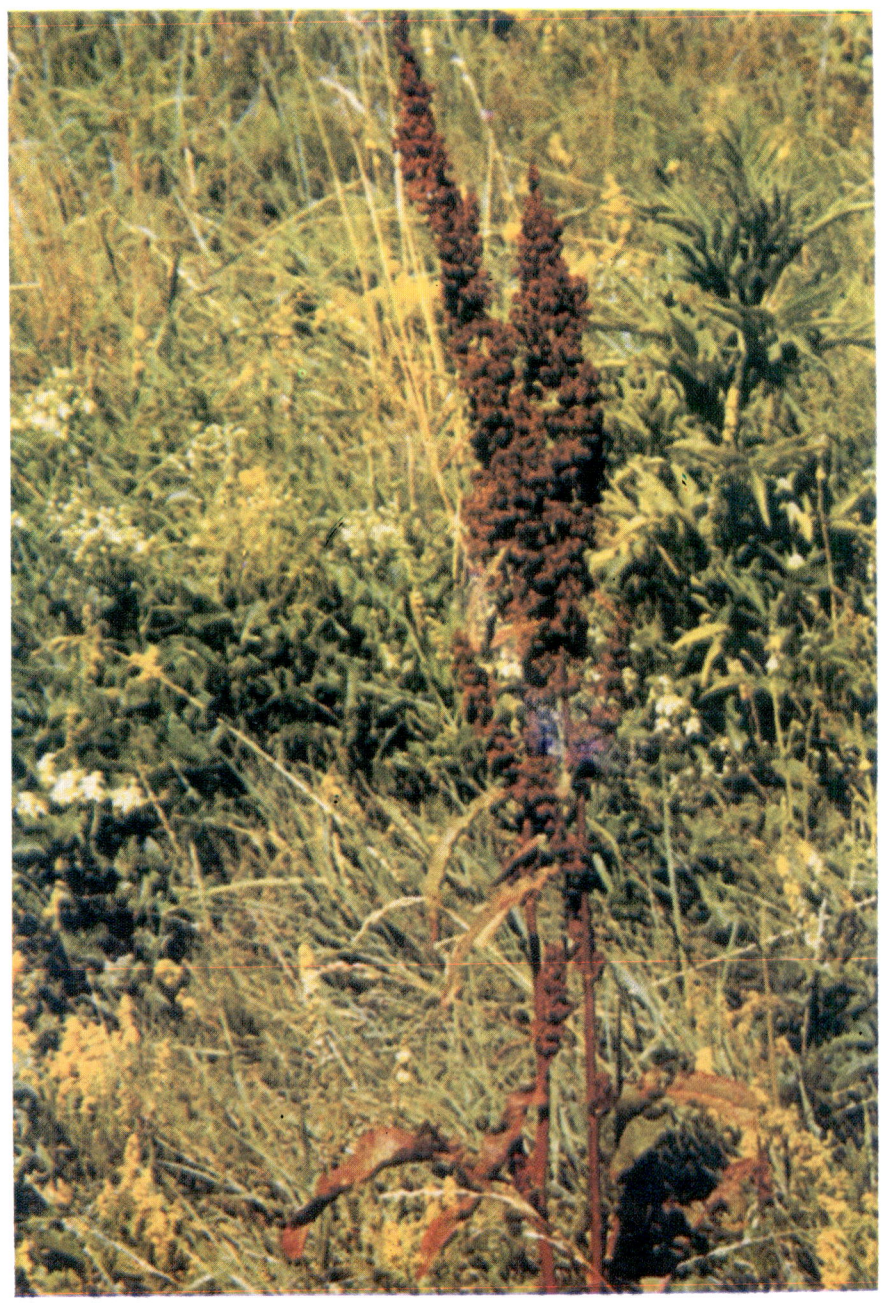

Rumex maritimus

(Courtesy : Dr. Peter Babulka, Budapest)

SCIENTIFIC NAME	:	*Rumex maritimus* Hook
UNANI NAME	:	JANGLI PALAK
FAMILY	:	*Polygonaceae*
PARTS USED	:	Whole plant, leaves

PHARMACOLOGICAL PROPERTIES RELEVANT TO THERAPEUTIC USE IN SKIN DISEASES

While the plant is claimed to be useful in skin diseases, some species of Rumex are considered poisonous and harmful to the skin. For example *R. acetosa* Linn, when taken in excess, may cause poisoning due to its high oxolic acid content while its leaves are reported to produce dermatitis. Other species e.g. *R. nepalensis* Spreng and *R. orientalis* Benth, on the other hand, are considered popular remedies against the ill effects of stinging nettles (e.g. *Urtica dioica* Linn). These bring relief when rubbed over the affected part. Fortunately these species are commonly found close to the nettles[174]. *R. maritimus* Hook is reported to contain some antifungal constituents[14]. Joglekar and Balwani[212] reported antipruritic activity in this plant. A 3% ointment made from the plant extracts brought about relief from *Mucuna pruriens* induced itching in dogs. Various species of *Rumex* are reported to contain substantial amounts of Vitamin C; the maximum content (750-1200 mg%) was observed in the dry leaves of *R. acetosella* Linn[25].

ELEMENTAL COMPOSITION[227]

Element	Concentration (mg/g ash)
Copper	0.195
Zinc	0.025
Iron	0.004
Manganese	0.020
Magnesium	3.100
Chromium	0.006
Nickel	0.039
Cadmium	0.001
Cobalt	0.004
Lead	0.002
Silver	0.001
Molybdenum	0.001
Tin	ND

ND : Not detected

SCIENTIFIC NAME	:	*Santalum album* Linn
UNANI	:	SANDAL SAFED
FAMILY	:	*Santaonaceae*
PARTS USED	:	Wood, volatile oil

PHARMACOLOGICAL PROPERTIES RELEVANT TO THEIRAPEUTIC USE IN SKIN DISEASES

It is attributed with blood purifying, soothing, refrigerant, antiseptic, astringent, antiinflammatory and insect repellent properties. The wood is ground with water to form a paste. This paste is applied to relieve itching in cases of erysepelas, prurigo, scabies, sudamina and inflammatory conditions of the skin[2,7,8,27,174]. Leaves are reported to contain phenolic constituents with antiviral activity. The oil is useful in urinary and respiratory tract infections and tuberculosis. It is reported to elicit antifungal effects also[7,213-216].

ELEMENTAL COMPOSITION[229]

Element	Concentration (mg/g ash)
Magnesium	71.875
Zinc	0.533
Iron	1.287
Calcium	494.485
Lead	0.037
Manganese	1.360
Copper	0.662
Nickel	0.156
Cobalt	ND
Mercury	Traces
Silver	ND
Strontium	Traces
Tin	Traces
Molybdenum	ND

ND : Not detected

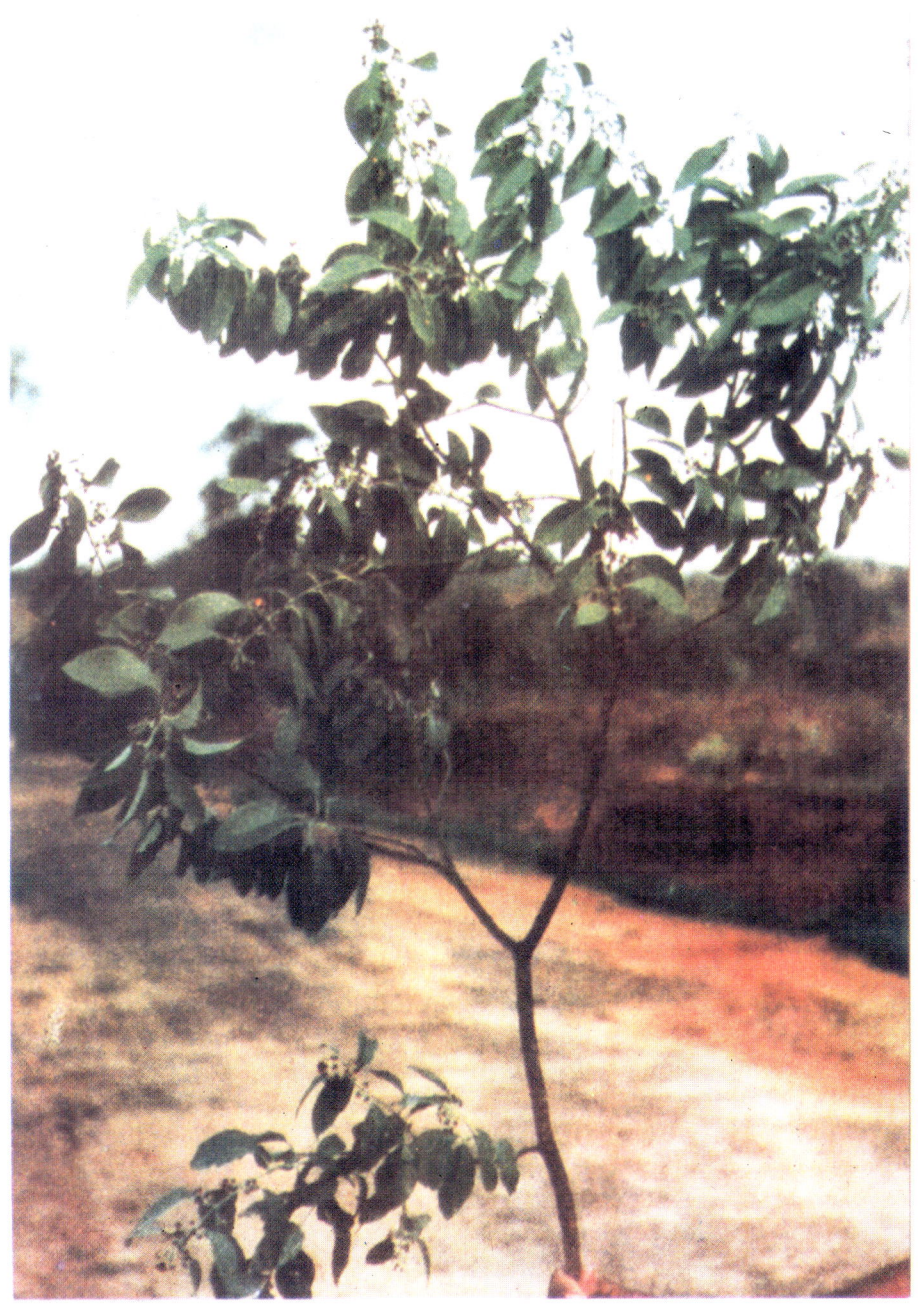

Santalum album
(Courtesy : C.C.R.U.M., New Delhi)

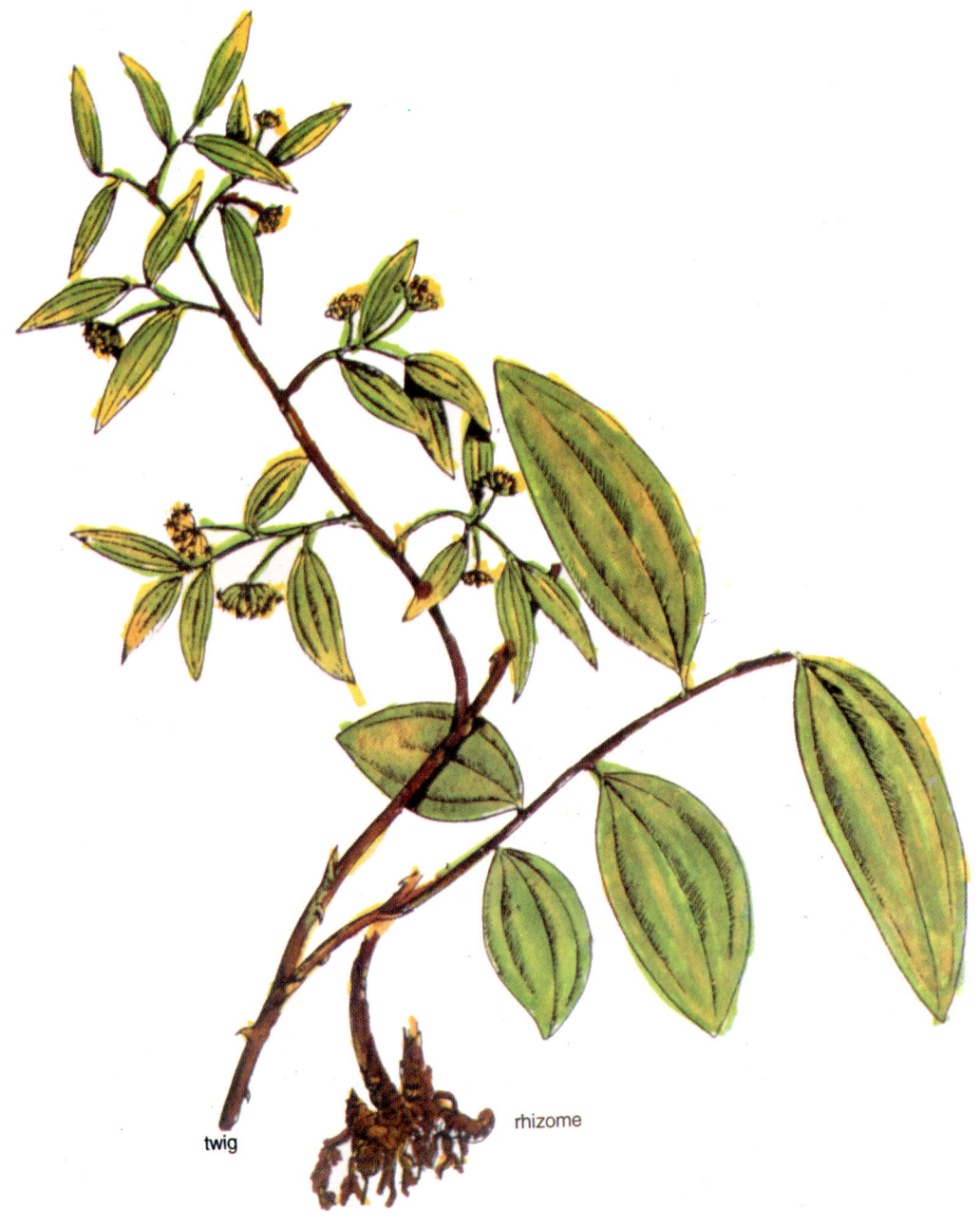

twig   rhizome

Smilax china

SCIENTIFIC NAME	:	*Smilax china* Linn
UNANI NAME	:	CHOBCHINI
FAMILY	:	*Liliaceae*
PARTS USED	:	Roots

PHARMACOLOGICAL PROPERTIES RELEVANT TO THERAPEUTIC USE IN SKIN DISEASES

The roots possess alterative, demulcent, tonic and blood purifying properties with claimed utility in skin diseases, chronic rheumatism, inflammatory conditions and syphilis[7,8,174]. No reports on scientific investigations are available.

ELEMENTAL COMPOSITION[228]

Element	Concentration (μg/g ash)
Copper	240.00
Zinc	50.00
Iron	5.38×10^3
Manganese	388.00
Magnesium	62.00×10^3
Chromium	12.40
Nickel	26.80
Tin	0.18
Molybdenum	50.40
Silver	0.94
Lead	380.00
Cobalt	10.60

ND - Not detected

SCIENTIFIC NAME	:	*Sphaeranthus indicus* Kurtz
UNANI NAME	:	MUNDI
FAMILY	:	*Compositae*
PARTS USED	:	Flowers, leaves roots and root bark

PHARMACOLOGICAL PROPERTIES RELEVANT TO THERAPEUTIC USE IN SKIN DISEASES

The plant is attributed with emollient, antiseptic, blood purifying, tonic, resolvent and styptic properties and are used in chronic skin diseases, urticaria, conjunctivitis, bleeding piles and for dispersion of tumours[2,7,8,27,174]. Ethanolic extract of flowers was investigated for its claimed hemostatic activity but it did not affect bleeding time, clotting time and prothrombin time in rabbits[217].

ELEMENTAL COMPOSITION OF FLOWERS[176]

Element	Concentration (mg/g ash)
Magnesium	12.132
Calcium	15.812
Lead	0.144
Copper	0.082
Mercury	ND
Cobalt	ND
Zinc	0.720
Iron	0.162
Chromium	Traces
Cadmium	ND
Manganese	0.123
Nickel	ND
Silver	ND
Molybdenum	ND

ND : Not detected

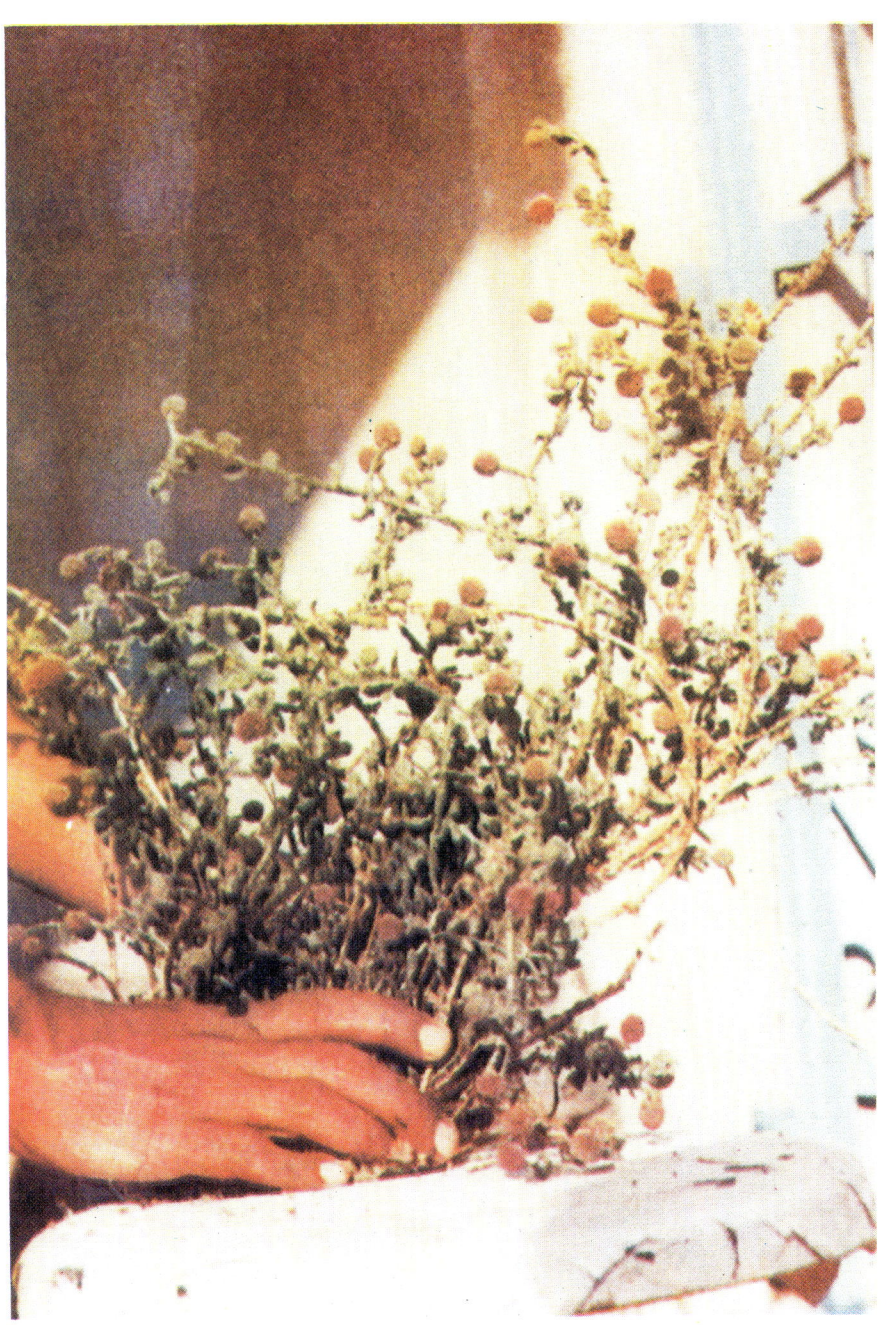

Sphaeranthus indicus

(Courtesy : C.C.R.U.M., New Delhi)

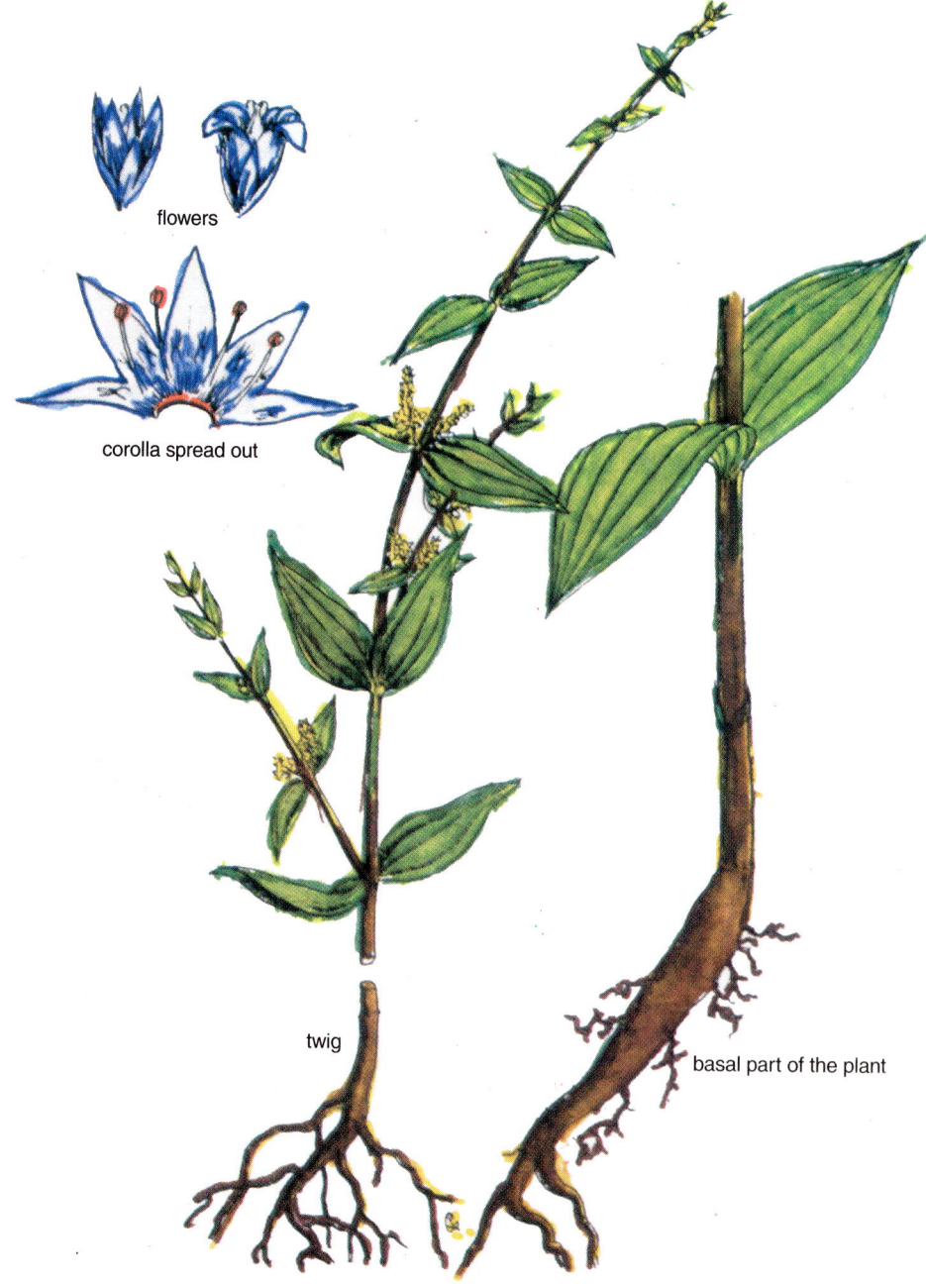

flowers

corolla spread out

twig

basal part of the plant

Swertia chirata
(Courtesy : Hamdard Dawakhana, Delhi)

SCIENTIFIC NAME	:	*Swertia chirata* Buch Ham
UNANI NAME	:	CHIRATA TALKH
FAMILY	:	*Gentinaceae*
PARTS USED	:	Whole plant

PHARMACOLOGICAL PROPERTIES RELEVANT TO THERAPEUTIC USE IN SKIN DISEASES

It is a reputed drug with claimed utility in various skin diseases including scabies, inflammatory conditions, eczema, leucoderma, scorpion sting, gout etc.[2,7,8,27,174]. Experimental and clinical studies carried out at the Skin Institute and Institute of Dermatology, New Delhi revealed its ability to promote phagocytic activity and efficacy in the treatment of patients of acne vulgaris sehorrhoeic folliculitis, chronic pyoderma, infective eczema and furunculosis[176].

ELEMENTAL COMPOSITION OF FLOWERS[176]

Element	Concentration (mg/g ash)
Magnesium	41.494
Calcium	26.971
Lead	0.301
Copper	0.109
Mercury	ND
Cobalt	ND
Zinc	1.063
Iron	0.194
Chromium	ND
Cadmium	Traces
Manganese	0.324
Nickel	ND
Silver	ND
Molybdenum	ND

ND : Not detected

SCIENTIFIC NAME	:	*Terminalia chebula* Retz
UNANI NAME	:	HALEELA SIYAH/HARAR
FAMILY	:	*Combretaceae*
PARTS USED	:	Fruits

PHARMACOLOGICAL PROPERTIES RELEVANT TO THERAPEUTIC USE IN SKIN DISEASES

While the unripe fruits are purgative, the ripe fruits possess antihistaminic, astringent and blood purifying properties. Infusion is useful in wounds, sores, bleeding ulcers, piles, leprosy, snake bite, scorpion sting and stomatitis[2,7,8,27,174,176]. Antibacterial, antifungal and mild antihistaminic actions have been confirmed in the plant by experimental investigations[156,157]. Antimicrobial properties were also reported in the crude extracts of another species (*T. belerica*)[5].

ELEMENTAL COMPOSITION OF FLOWERS[176,228]

Elements	Concentration (mg/g ash)
Magnesium	29.752
Calcium	33.346
Lead	0.139
Copper	0.107
Mercury	ND
Cobalt	0.002
Zinc	0.597
Iron	0.209
Chromium	ND
Cadmium	Traces
Manganese	0.099
Nickel	ND
Silver	0.003
Molybdenum	0.001
Tin	ND

ND : Not detected

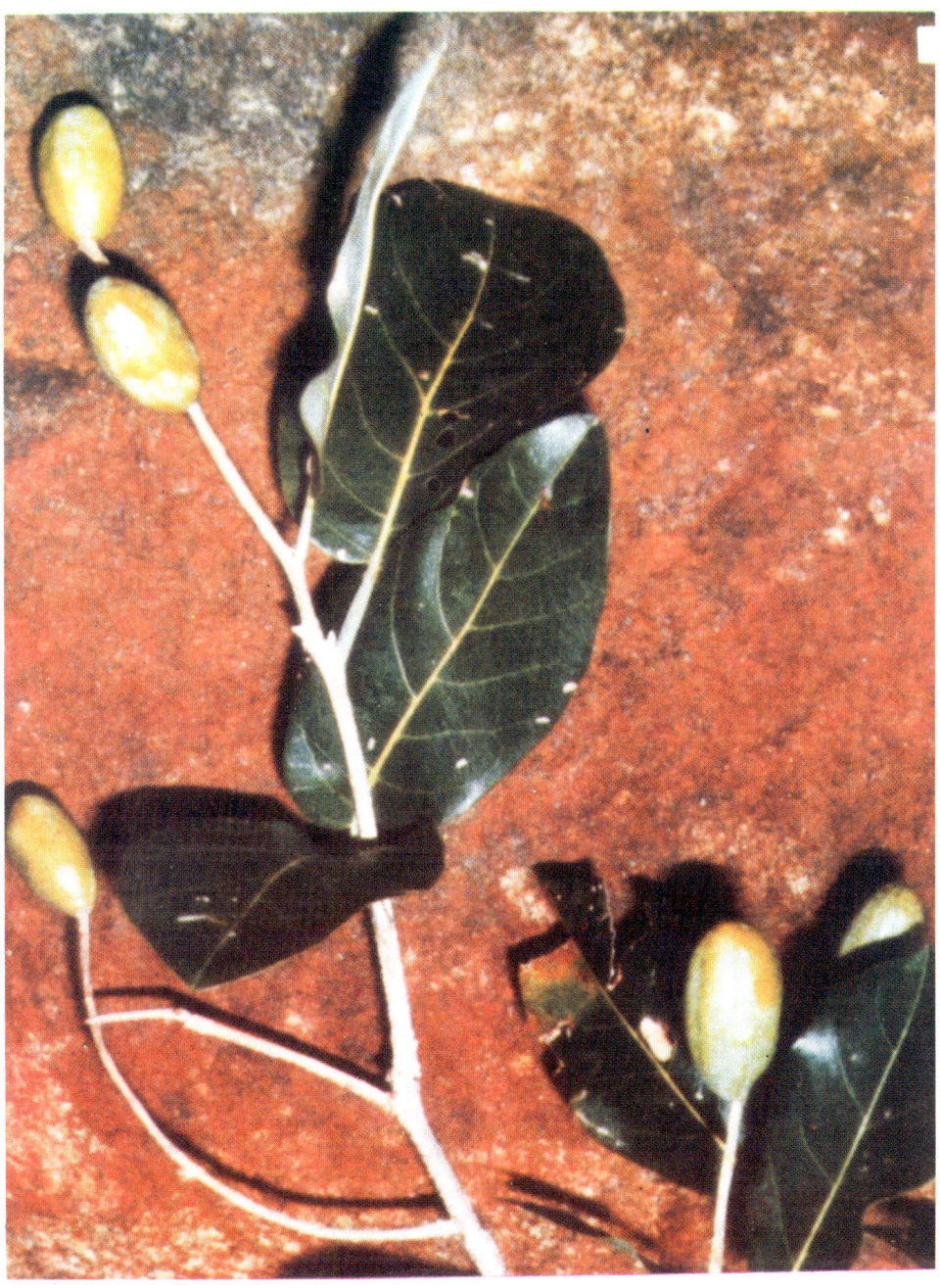

Terminalia chebula

(Field Photo : Dr. M.P. Sharma and Mr. Kaiser N. Khan)

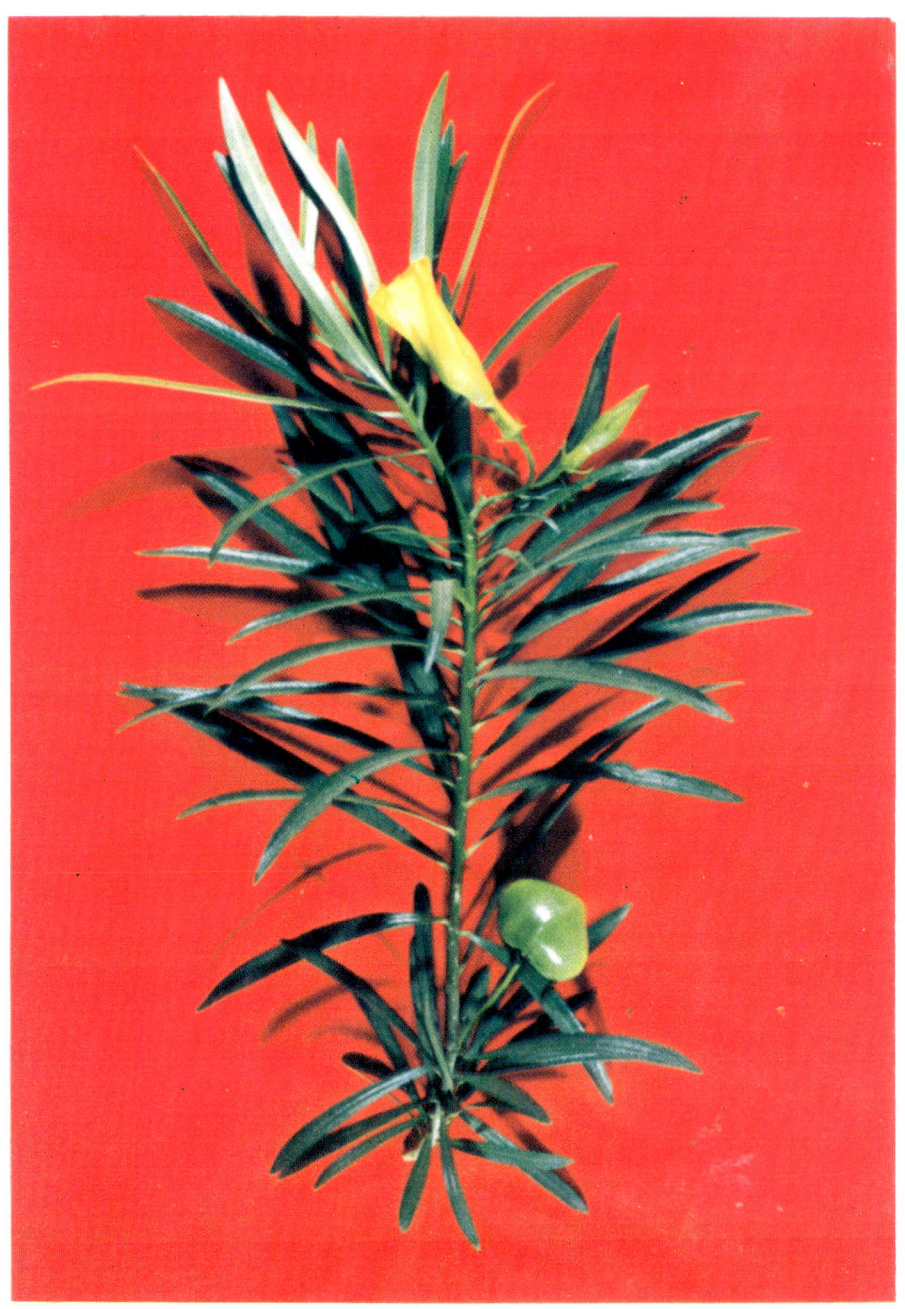

Thevetia neriifolia

(Field Photo : Dr. M.P. Sharma and Mr. Kaiser N. Khan)

SCIENTIFIC NAME	:	*Thevetia neriifolia* Juss
UNANI NAME	:	KANER ZARD
FAMILY	:	*Apocyanaceae*
PARTS USED	:	Bark, seeds and leaves

PHARMACOLOGICAL PROPERTIES RELEVANT TO THERAPEUTIC USE IN SKIN DISEASES

Though the plant is reputed for its cardiac glycosides, its use has also been mentioned for the treatment of skin diseases[7]. No scientific reports are, however, available.

ELEMENTAL COMPOSITION OF LEAVES[227, 228]

Elements	Concentration (mg/g ash)
Copper	0.167
Zinc	0.145
Iron	0.05
Manganese	0.209
Magnesium	66.000
Chromium	0.077
Nickel	0.013
Cadmium	ND
Cobalt	0.007
Lead	0.017
Silver	0.001
Molybdenum	0.011
Tin	0.0001

ND : Not detected

SCIENTIFIC NAME	:	*Tinospora cordifolia* Miers
UNANI NAME	:	GILOE
FAMILY	:	*Menispermaceae*
PARTS USED	:	Stem and roots

PHARMACOLOGICAL PROPERTIES RELEVANT TO THERAPEUTIC USE IN SKIN DISEASES

The plant is attributed with blood purifying, detoxicant, alterative, febrifuge and antirheumatic properties with claimed utility in the treatment of inflammatory conditions, skin diseases, snake bite and scorpion sting cases, syphilis and gonorrhoea[2,7,8,27]. Antiinflammatory activity was confirmed by experimental studies using a variety of models including oedema induced by formalin, carrageenin, yeast, egg albumin, terpentine, and serotonin; arthritis induced by Freund's adjuvant; granuloma induced by croton oil and cotton pellet; and effects on histamine and serotonin content of skin. These were reviewed by Vohora and Wani[28].

ELEMENTAL COMPOSITION[227]

Element	Concentration (mg/g ash)
Magnesium	24.518
Calcium	42.665
Lead	0.147
Copper	0.088
Mercury	0.167
Cobalt	0.022
Zinc	0.765
Iron	0.440
Chromium	ND
Cadmium	Traces
Manganese	0.083
Nickel	ND
Silver	0.001
Molybdenum	0.018
Tin	0.0002

ND : Not detected

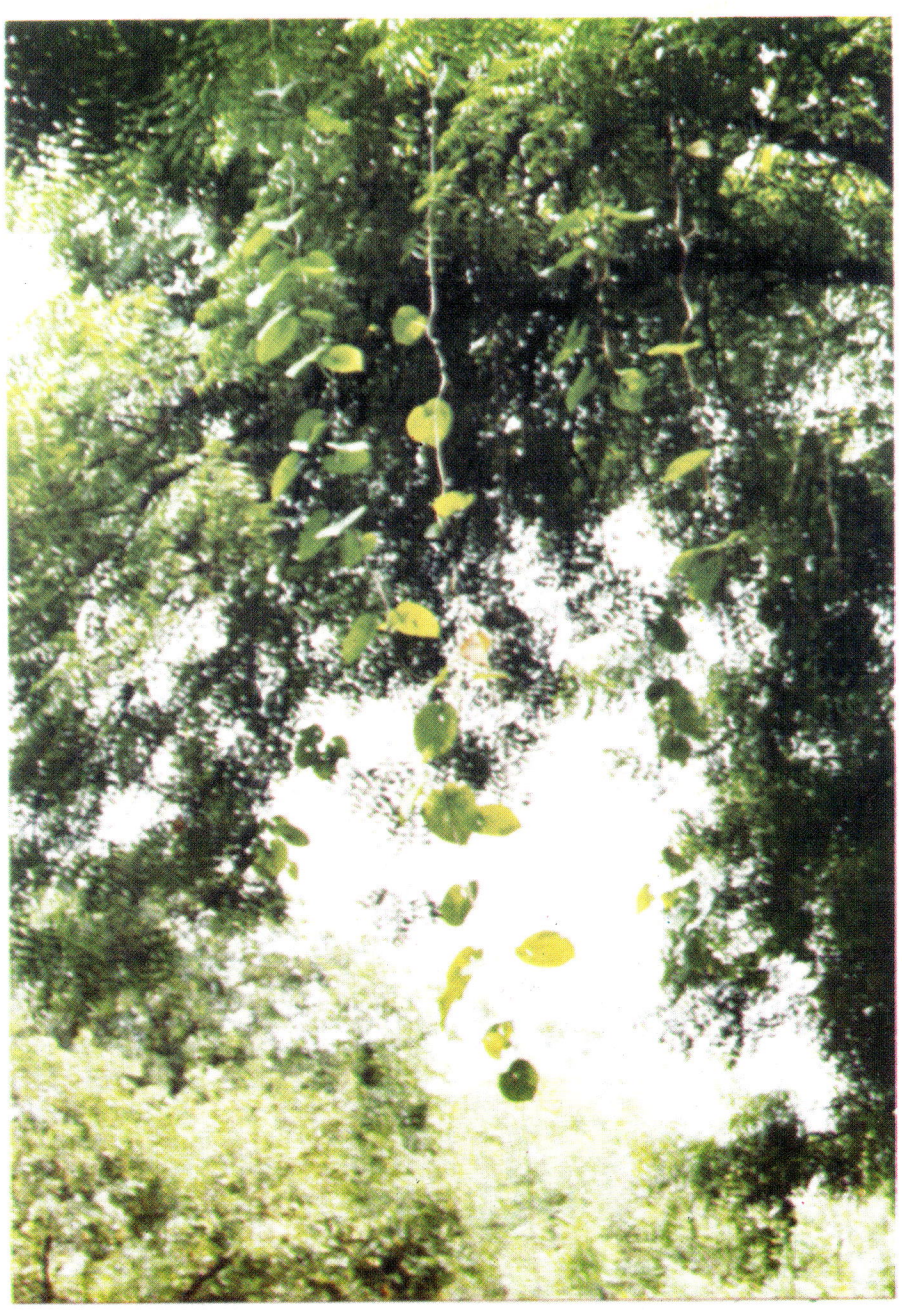

Tinospora cordifolia

(Field Photo : Dr. M.P. Sharma and Mr. Kaiser N. Khan)

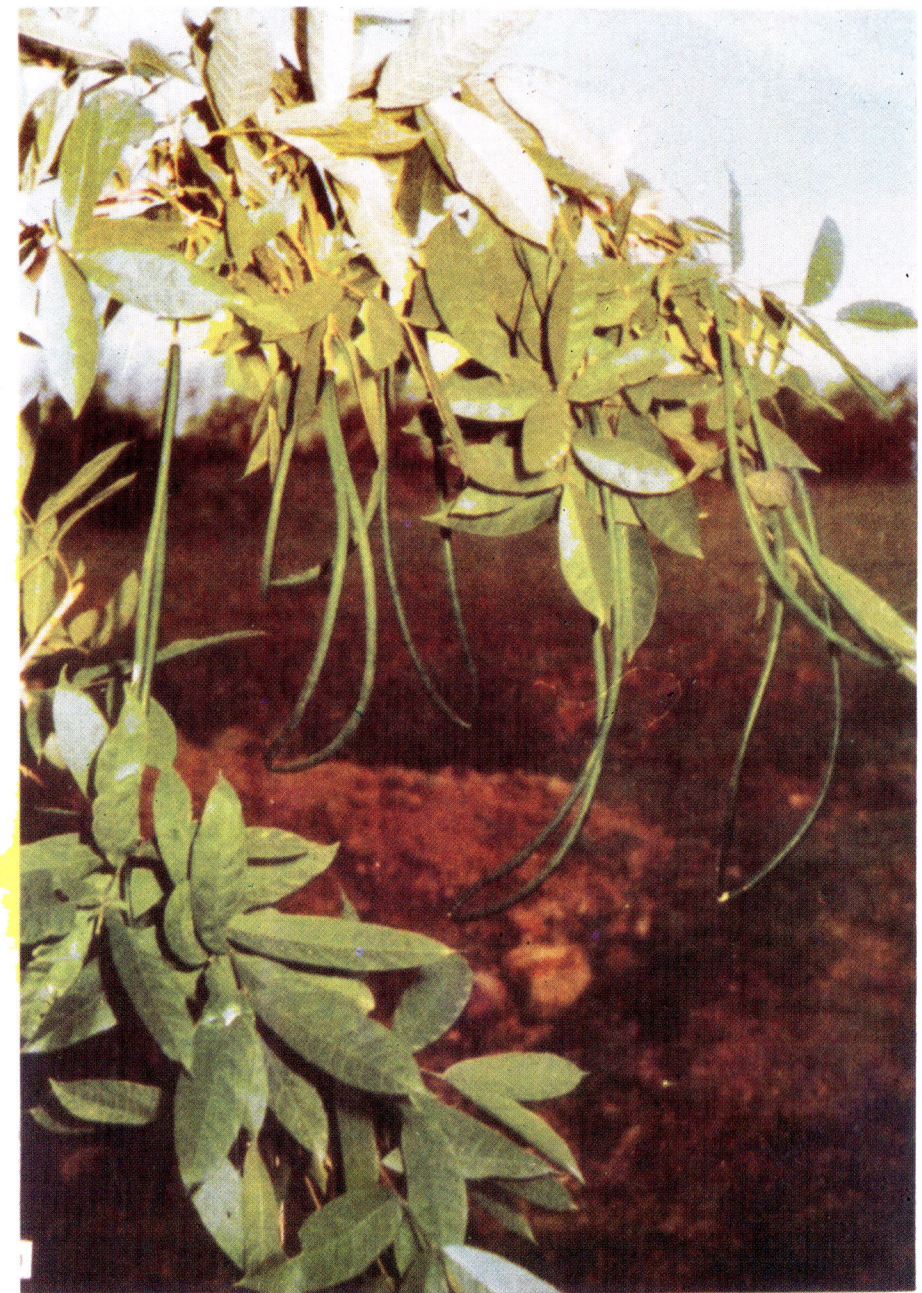

Wrightia tinctoria

(Courtesy : C.C.R.U.M., New Delhi)

| SCIENTIFIC NAME | : | *Wrightia tinctoria* Br |
| SCIENTIFIC NAME | : | *Wrightia tinctoria* Br |

SCIENTIFIC NAME : *Wrightia tinctoria* Br

UNANI NAME : INDERJOU SHIREEN

FAMILY : *Apocyanaceae*

PARTS USED : Whole plant

PHARMACOLOGICAL PROPERTIES RELEVANT TO THERAPEUTIC USE IN SKIN DISEASES

The plant is claimed to possess antiseptic and antimicrobial properties (including antitubercular action) and is used for the treatment of various skin diseases[174]. In a screening programme carried out at the Central Drug Research Institute, Lucknow an ethanolic extract of the whole plant without roots exhibited anticancer activity[21].

ELEMENTAL COMPOSITION[176]

Element	Concentration (mg/g ash)
Copper	0.281
Zinc	0.017
Iron	0.0004
Manganese	0.046
Magnesium	0.003
Chromium	0.002
Nickel	0.053
Cadmium	0.0006

ND : Not Detected

SCIENTIFIC NAME	:	Zingiber zerumbet Rosc
UNANI NAME	:	·NARKACHOOR
FAMILY	:	*Zingiberaceae*
PARTS USED	:	Rhizomes

PHARMACOLOGICAL PROPERTIES RELEVANT TO THERAPEUTIC USE IN SKIN DISEASES

It is attributed with antiseptic and blood purifying properties and is claimed to be useful for treating various skin diseases including leprosy[174,176]. Antibacterial activity was confirmed by experimental studies on a sesquiterpene lactone isolated from the plant[166]. Other species of *Zingiber* (e.g. *Z. officinalis*, *Z. capticum*) are reported to elicit antibacterial, antiviral and anti-cancer effects[14,21].

ELEMENTAL COMPOSITION[176]

Element	Concentration (mg/g ash)
Magnesium	20.74
Calcium	9.26
Lead	ND
Copper	0.04
Mercury	0.07
Cobalt	ND
Zinc	0.63
Iron	0.31
Chromium	ND
Cadmium	ND
Manganese	0.09
Nickel	ND
Silver	ND
Molybdenum	ND

ND : Not detected

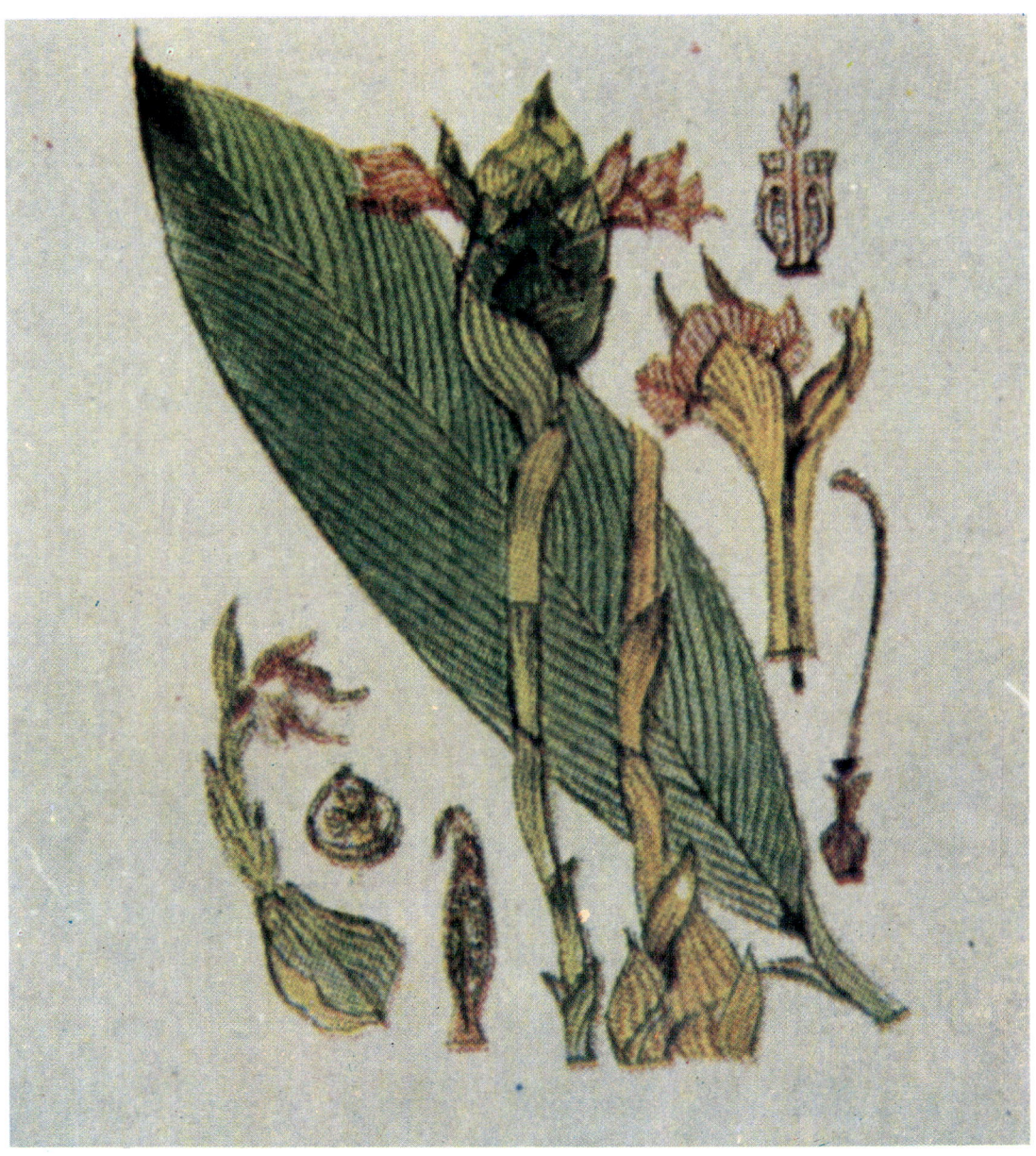

Zingiber zerumbet
(Courtesy : Hamdard Dawakhana, Delhi)

4.4 FORMULATIONS

Single drugs are rarely used in Indian systems of medicine; mostly multi-ingredient formulations are used for therapy with twin purposes of synergistic action of different components and reduction of toxic side effects. Several reports are available on the clinical efficacy of such formulations in various skin diseases. These include some coded drugs of the Central Council for Research in Unani Medicine e.g. $BSL_5 + BS_4$ and $BS_9 + BS_{10}$ for leucoderma, $NF_1 + NFL_2$ for eczema and $NF_1 + NFL_3$ for dermatitis[218]. Similar reports are available for many Ayurvedic and Siddha formulations which include some coded drugs of the Central Council for Ayurveda and Siddha e.g. Shashikala Vati, CRIA-9 and Ayush-57 for leucoderma, Chandamutham for psoriasis, Chop Chingadi Mishran for itching, and the following drug schedule for the treatment of skin diseases in general[219].

(a)	Gandhak Rasayana Arogyawardhini Manjistha Churna	}	Combination
(b)	Patoladi kwath Khadiraristha	}	as Anupana
(c)	Triphala Churna		
(d)	Nimba Tail Nimba Kwath	}	for external use

Zafarulla and coworkers[220] reviewed Unani formulations mentioned in ancient texts for the treatment of leprosy (Please see Chapter 7, Table 7.4).

Safi, a popular blood purifying formulation used in the Indian subcontinent for improving complexion and treatment of acne, pimples and blemishes, has been extensively investigated. It was found to elicit anti-bacterial and antifungal activity against *Staphylococcus aureus, Bacillus subtilis, Streptococcus pyogenes, Aspergillus flavus, Aspergillus nigra, Aspergillus fermigatus, Trichophyton rubrum* and *Trichocphyton mentagrophytes*. Oral administration of the formulation for one week was shown to enhance the protective immune response. It caused activation of the macrophages of the reticular endothelial system as evidenced by accelerated clearance rate of colloidal carbon from the test system. It increased cell mediated immune response. The effects were studied on an immunocompetant system (T cells, B cells and macrophages) using the parameters: erythrocyte rosette, delayed type hypersensitivity and serum antibody levels with very encouraging results. Further clinical efficacy was reported in cases of acne, eczema, psoriasis, impetigo tinea, tinea versicolor, ringworm and leucoderma. One of the important metabolic pathways in cutaneous biochemistry linked with proliferation of epidermal cells are polyamines derived from the amino acid orinthine. An interesting finding was that cutaneous ornithine decarboxylase enzyme levels decreased in patients of impetigo and tinea following treatment with this formulation[221]. A survey of literature showed that the constituent plants of this formulation possess antibacterial, antifungal, antiviral, diuretic, antiallergic/antihistaminic, choleretic, hypoglycemic, hypocholesterolemic, and antiinflammatory properties which were equated to its claimed blood purifying effects in Unani medicine[176,222]. Safety evaluation studies carried out on human volunteers at the Clinical Pharmacology Centre of Grant Medical College, Bombay using biochemical, physical and subjective parameters, revealed that the formulation was well tolerated and showed no adverse effects[221].

Since acne occur in young adults and more commonly in females, the presence of sugar in *Safi* possibly has an adverse influence on its acceptibility. This prompted Dr. R.D. Kulkarni, Emeritus Professor at the Department of Pharmacology, MGM Medical College, Mumbai, to undertake a clinical investigation using a tablet formulation of *Safi*. This open non-competitive self control study exhibited marked beneficial effect in acne. Of the 40 patients, receiving two tablets twice a day, 11 had complete clearance of the lesions after only 2 weeks of therapy and another 19 patients showed similar effect at the end of 4 weeks. Of the remaining 10 patients, 8 were shifted to the lowest grade of disease (grade I) indicating considerable improvement. Besides the mean lesion count showed progressive decline. Thus only 2/40 patients (one each in grade II and III) can be considered refractory to treatment. Both these patients had lesions for over 6 months suggesting chronicity of lesions as the cause for failure in these cases. There were no adverse effects.

Clinical studies on herbomineral tablets (containing Chaksu, Narkachur, Karanj, Reetha, Katha safed, Indrayan, Zinc sulphate and Magnesium sulphate) given orally and an oil (containing Roghan Kamela, *Ammi majus*, Salicyclic acid, Roghan and Tarcoal) used by local application, yielded interesting results in cases of psoriasis. The formulations were prepared by one of the authors (Abdul Hameed) and investigations were carried by scientists of the Skin Institute and School of Dermatology, New Delhi. Of the 53 patients of psoriasis, on this therapeutic regimen, the frequency distribution of % improvement (vs number of patients) was as follows: 100% (5), 76-99% (6), 51-75% (8), 26-50% (12) and < 25% (22).

Another study by the same group revealed encouraging results in cases of acne. Of the 59 patients, treated with herbomineral tablets (containing Safoof safi, Neem extract, Amla, Karanj, Yeast and Zinc sulphate), the % improvement (vs number of patients) was as follows: 100% (10), 76-99% (2), 51-75% (9), 25-50% (8), < 25% (24). Six patients, under this study, were irregular and showed poor compliance.

Clinical studies on some formulations for use in other skin diseases including eczema, scabies and air borne contact dermatitis are in progress. The preliminary findings appear to be promising but the data available so far is insufficient for definite conclusions.

REFERENCES

1. Vohora SB, Babulka P, Botz L et al. (1987) *Curare*, Germany **10**, 249.
2. Behl BN, Arora RB and Srivastava G (1992) *Traditional Indian Dermatology*, New Delhi: Skin Institute and School of Dermatology.
3. Satyavati GV, Raina MK and Sharma M (1976) *Medicinal Plants of India*, vol 1, pp. 114-116, 458-466,New Delhi. Indian Council of Medical Research
4. Desai VB and Sirsi M (1966) *Indian J Med Res* **28**, 164.
5. Naqvi SAH, Khan MSY and Vohora SB (1990) *Fitoterapia*, Italy **52(3)**, 221.
6. Bhakuni DS, Dhar ML, Dhar MM et al (1971) *Indian J Exp Biol* **9**, 91.
7. *National Seminar on Use of Medicinal Plants in Skin Care* (1994). Lucknow: Central Institute of Medicinal and Aromatic Plants.
8. Wahid A and Siddiqui HH (1961) *A Survey of Drugs*, ed 2, pp. 118, 119, 140, 141, 148, 154, 155, 159-161, New Delhi: Institute of History of Medicine and Medical Research.
9. Dhar ML, Dhar MM, Dhawan BN et al (1968) *Indian J Exp Biol* **6**, 232.

10. Joshi CG and Magar NG (1952) *J Sci Industr Res* **11B(6)**, 261.

11. Singh L. and Sharma M (1978) *Geobios* **5(2)**, 99.

12. Singhal PC and Joshi LD (1984) *Current Sci.* **53(2)**, 91.

13. Srimal SK (1980) *Biol Abstr* **69(1)**, 512, No. 4086.

14. Satyavati GV (1984) In: *Current Research in Pharmacology in India* (eds Das PK and Dhawan BN), pp.119-146, New Delhi: Indian National Science Academy.

15. Dhawan BN, Patnaik GK,Rastogi RP et al (1977) *Indian J Exp Biol* **15**, 208.

16. Jain SR and Kar A (1971) *Planta Medica* **20**, 118.

17. Bhakuni DS, Goel AK, Jain S et al (1990) *Indian J Exp Biol* **28**, 619.

18. Gokhle SD and Karandikar GK (1960) *Indian J Pharm* **22(11)**, 278.

19. Chakraborti SK and Mukerji B (1968) *J Res Indian Med* **3(1)**, 70.

20. Singh RH, Khosla RL and Upadhyaya BB (1974) *J Res Indian Med* **9(2)**, 65.

21. Rastogi RP and Dhawan BN (1982) *Indian J Med Res* **76 Suppl**, 27.

22. Bedi R (1968) *Ayurved Mahasammelan Patrika* **55**, 35.

23. Prasad BN (1962) *Leprosy Rev* **33**, 207.

24. Patel RP and Alex RM (1967) *Indian J Med Sci* **21**, 229.

25. Siddiqui TO and Ahmad J (1985) *Indian Drugs* **23(2)**, 1.

26. Gujral ML, Saxena PN and Mishra SS (1955) *J Indian Med Ass* **25(2)**, 49.

27. Kapoor LD (1990) *Handbook of Ayurvedic Medicinal Plants*, Boca Raton, Florida: CRC Press.

28. Vohora SB and Wani H (1987) *Herba Hungarica*, **26(1)**, 73.

29. Pal S., Chakravarty SK, Banerjee A et al (1968) *Indian J Med Res* **56(4)**, 445.

30. Bhatia VN (1970) *J Commun Dis* **2**, 38.

31. Dhar ML, Dhar MM, Dhawan BN et al (1973) *Indian J Exp Biol* **11**, 43.

32. Bhargava AK and Chouhan CS (1968) *Indian J Pharm* **30**, 150.

33. Dhar ML, Dhawan BN, Prasad CR et al (1974) *Indian J Exp Biol* **12**, 512.

34. Bhatnagar SS (1961) *Indian J Med Res* **49(5)**, 799.

35. Hemadri K and Rao SS (1984) *Ancient Sci Life* **3(4)**, 209.

36. Mukherjee GD (1976) *J Res Indian Med* **11(2)**, 66.

37. Nigam P, Kapoor KK,Gupta AK et al (1958) *Med & Surg* **22(6)**, 13.

38. Bhakuni DS, Dhar ML, Dhar MM et al (1969) *Indian J Exp Biol* **7**, 250.

39. Naqvi SAH, Khan MSY and Vohora SB (1976) *Planta Medica*, Germany **29**, 98.

40. Lalithakumari H, Sirsi M and Govindrajan VS (1965) *Indian J Exp Biol* **3**, 66.

41. Dhawan BN, Dubey MP, Mehrotra BN et al (1980) *Indian J Exp Biol* **18**, 594.

42. Patel RP and Trivedi BM (1957) *Indian J Med Sci* **11**, 887.

43. Venkitaraman S and Radhakrishnan N (1972) *Indian J Pharmacol* **4**, 148.

44. Chopra IC, Gupta KC and Nazir BN (1952) *Indian J Med Res* **40**, 511.

45. Rao AR (1969) *Indian J Med Res* **57**, 459.

46. Dutta NK and Panse MV (1962) *Indian J Med Res*, **50**, 732.

47. Dutta NK and Natrajan Iyer S (1968) *Indian J Med Res* **50**, 349.

48. Amin AH, Subbaiah TV and Abbasi KM (1969) *Canad J Microbiol* **15**, 1067.

49. Godbole SH and Pendse GS (1960) *Indian J Pharm* **22(2)**, 89.

50. Gujral ML and Saxena PN (1956) *Indian J Med Res* **44**, 657.

51. Godhwani JL, Vyas DS and Godhwani S (1985) *Indian J Pharmacol* **17** suppl-1 Abst p. 36.

52. Kar A and Jain SR (1971) *Qualitas Plantes Mater Veg* **20**, 231.

53. Neogi NC and NayakKP (1958) *Indian J Pharm* **20**, 95.

54. George M. Venkataraman PR and Prandalai KM (1947) *J Sci Indistr Res* **6B(3)**, 42.

55. Iyengar MA and Pendse GS (1965) *Indian J Pharm* **27**, 307.

56. Krishnarao RV and Reddy NR (1977) *Indian J Pharm* **36(6)**, 165.

57. Marilangan VA (1959) *Phllipp J Sci* **88(2)**, 245.

58. Singh RN (1971) *Labdev J Sci Tech* **9B(2)**, 136.

59. Radhakrishnan Potti G and Kurup PA (1970) *Indian J Exp Biol* **8**, 39.

60. Shukla DP and Murty CRK (1961) *J Sci Industr Res* **20C**, 109.

61. Juneja JR, Gaind KN and Panesar AS (1970) *Res Bull Punjab Univ* **21**, 519.

62. Gaind KN, Juneja JR and Jain PC (1969) *Indian J Pharm* **31**, 24.

63. Patel RP and Patel KC (1956) *Indian J Pharm* **18**, 107.

64. Lillikutty J and Santhakumari G (1969) *J Res Indian Med* **4**, 25.

65. Gaind KN, Juneja TR and Bhandarkar PN (1972) *Indian J Pharm* **34**, 86.

66. Shukla SD, Modi TN and Deshmankar BS (1973) *Indian J Pharm* **35**, 40.

67. Patel RP and Patel KD (1957) *Indian J Pharm* **19**, 70.

68. Rao VR and Gupta I (1971) *Indian J Pharmacol* **3**, 29.

69. Pal S and Gupta I (1971) *Indian J Pharmacol* **3**, 29.

70. Patel RP and Trivedi BM (1962) *Indian J Med Res* **50**, 218.

71. Seth UKand Setty VH (1970) In: *Advances in Research in Indian Medicine* (eds Udupa KN, Chaturvedi GN and Tripathi SN), pp. 1-55, Varanasi: Banaras Hindu University.

72. Seth UK, Vaz A. Delliwala CV et al (1963) *Arch Int Pharmacodyn* **114(1,2)**, 34.

73. Singh N, Chand N and Kohli RP (1974) *J Res Indian Med* **9(1)**, 7.

74. Jindal MN, Patel VK and Patel NB (1975) *Indian J Pharmacol* **71(1,2)**, 104.

75. Gaind KN, Chopra BM and Kaul RN (1965) *Indian J Pharm* **27**, 262.

76. Ramaswamy AS, Jayaraman S and Sirsi M et al (1972) *Indian J Exp Biol* **10**, 72.

77. Khonde PA, SrivastavaPN and Ahmad A (1971) *Indian J Pharmacol* **3**, 20.

78. Singh H and Ghosh MN (1968) *Indian J Physiol Pharmacol***12**, 22.

79. Singh H and Ghosh MN (1976) *Indian J Physiol Pharmacol***14**, 57.

80. Singh H and Ghosh MN (1972) *Indian J Pharmacol* **4**, 151.

81. Acharya BK, Modi ML and Sinha SN (1964) *J Indian Med Asso* **33**, 592.

82. Arora RB, Basu N and Jain AP (1970) *Second Indo-Soviet Sympo Chem Nat Prods including Pharmacol*, New Delhi, p. 133.

83. Banerjee A and Nigam SS (1978) *J Res Indian Med* **13(2)**, 63.

84. Basu AP (1971) *Indian J Pharm* **33(6)**, 127.

85. Bhatia A,Singh BG and Khanna NM (1964) *Indian J Exp Biol* **2**, 158.

86. Dinesh Chandra and Gupta SS (1972) *Indian J Med Res* **60**, 138.

87. Ghatak N and Basu N (1972) *Indian J Exp Biol* **10**, 235.

88. Gupta SS, Dineshchandra and Mishra N (1972) *Indian J Physiol Pharmacol* **16**, 264.

89. Pachauri SP and Mukherjee SK (1970) *J Res Indian Med* **5(1)**, 27.

90. Ramprasad C and Sirsi M (1956) *J Sci Industr Res* **15C**, 108.

91. Ramprasad C and Sirsi M (1967) *J Sci Industr Res* **16C**, 108.

92. Rao TS, Basu N and Siddiqui HH (1982) *Indian J Med Res* **75**, 574.

93. Rathore RS, Prakash A, Bhattacharya SK et al (1973) *Aspects Allergy Appl Immunol* **4**, 141.

94. Srimal RC, Khanna MM and Dhawan BN (1971) *Indian J Pharmacol* **8**, 10.

95. Victor G (1972) *Antiseptic* **69**, 163.

96. Yegnaryan R. Saraf AP and Balwani JH (1976) *Indian J Med Res* **64**, 601.

97. Patil JN and Srinivasan M (1971) *Indian J Exp Biol* **9**, 167.

98. De Lima OG (1963) *Biol Abstr* **44(6)**, 1877, Abstr no. 25212.

99. Jain PK (1979) *Indian Drugs* **16(6)**, 122

100. Anonymous (1952, 1956, 1972) *Wealth of India: Raw Materials* vol 3, p. 11; vol 4, p. 68, vol 9, p. 4, New Delhi: Council of Scientific and Industrial Research.

101. Gautam MP and Purohit RM(1973) *Indian J Pharm* **35**, 93.

102. Sanzgiri R and Nasir MNF (1969) *Bombay Hosp J* **11**, 167.

103. Patel RP, Shah CS, Khanna PN et al (1964) *Indian J Pharm* **26**, 168.

104. Khanna P and Nag TN (1973) *Indian J Pharm* **35**, 23.

105. Dutta NK, Dave KH, Desai SM et al (1968) *Indian J Med Res* **50**, 349.

106. Rama Rao SG, Subramanyam K, and Balasundaram D (1973) *Indian J Pharmacol* **5**, 258.

107. Anonymous (1966) *Eastern Pharmacist* **9(100)**, 107.

108. Nageshwara Rao KV and Narsingha Rao PL (1967) *Indian J Exp Biol* **5**, 96.

109. Nageshwara Rao KV and Narsimha Rao PL (1967) *Indian J Exp Biol* **5**, 101.

110. Santhanam K and Narsimha Rao PL (1968) *Indian J Exp Biol* **6**, 158.

111. Santhanam K and Narsimha Rao PL (1969) *Indian J Exp Biol* **7**, 34.

112. Verma SCL and Narsimha Rao PL (1967) *Indian J Exp Biol* **5**, 106.

113. Babbar OP, Choudhary BL, Singh MP et al (1970) *Indian J Exp Biol* **8**, 304.

114. Patel RN (1968) *Indian J Pharm* **30**, 43.

115. Khare AK, Srivastava MC and Tiwari JP (1982) *Indian Drugs* **19(6)**, 224.

116. Husain SMS, Singh DP, Saleem Y et al (1976) *J Res Indian Med* **11(2)**, 84.

117. Bajpai HS, Ojha JK and Singh RS (1971) *J Res Indian Med* **6(1)**, 1.

118. Bhat JB and Borker R (1953) *J Sci Industr Res* **12B**, 540.

119. Bhide NK, Mehta DJ, Attaker WW et al(1958) *Indian J Med Sci* **12**, 141.

120. Murty KS, Rao DN, Rao D et al (1978) *Indian J Pharmacol* **10(3)**, 247.

121. Murty SP and Sirsi M (1957) Lucknow: *Symposium Utilization Indian Medicinal Plants.*

122. Murty SP and Sirsi M (1958) *Indian J Physiol Pharmacol* **2**, 456.

123. Naryana DS (1965) *Mediscope* **8**, 322.

124. Pillai NR and Santhakumari G (1981) *Planta Medica* **43(1)**, 59.

125. Shah PM, Shah MJ, Sheth UK et al (1959) *J Asso Physns India* **7**, 235.

126. Shah PM, Sheth UK, Bhide NK et al (1958) *Indian J Med Sci* **12**, 150.

127. Singh N and Sastry MS (1981) *Indian J Pharmacol* **13(1)**, 102.

128. Thaker AM and Anjaria JV (1986) *Indian J Pharmacol* **18(3)**, 171.

129. Sanyal A and Verma KC (1969) *Indian J Microbiol* **9**, 23.

130. Raghunandan Rao R and George M (1949) *Indian J Med Res* **37**, 159.

131. Das BNR, Kurup PA, Narsimha Rao PL et al (1957) *Indian J Med Res* **45**, 197.

132. Lizzy KS, Narsimha Rao PL and Puthuswamy TL (1968) *Indian J Exp Biol* **6**, 168.

133. Agarwal OP (1972) *Indian J Pharm* **4**, 153.

134. Arora RB (1965) *Comparative Pharmacotherapeutics of Six Medicinal Plants Indigenous to India* HNF Monograph Series No. 1, pp. 44-45, New Delhi: Hamdard National Foundation.

135. Grover GS and Rao JT (1977) *Perfum Kosmet* **58(11)**, 328.

136. Jalil A (1971) *J Res Indian Med* **4**, 238.

137. Krishnamurty TR (1959) *Indian J Physiol Pharmacol* **3(2)**, 92.

138. Matsubhiro A and Nakada D (1955) *Antibiot Chemother* **5**, 22.

139. Venkitarman S and Gopalakrishnan N (1972) *Indian J Physiol Pharmacol* **16**, 265.

140. Vohora SB. Kumar I and Naqvi SAH (1972) *Indian J Pharm* **34**, 17.

141. Banger GP and Verma KC (1966) *Indian J Pharm* **28**, 77.

142. Tewari A, Sen SP and Guru LV (1966) *Indian Med Gaz* **6**, 22.

143. Gupta V, Bhatia VN Venugopal P et al (1971) *Indian J Med Res* **59**, 1002.

144. Anand KK, Sharma ML and Singh B (1978) *Indian J Exp Biol* **16(11)**, 1126.

145. Gaind KN, Dhar RN and Kaul RN (1965) *Indian J Pharm* **26**, 141.

146. Gaind KN, Dhar RN and Kaul RN (1965) *J Pharm Sci* **53**,1428.

147. Gupta KC, Bhatia MC and Chopra CL (1962) *Bull RRL Jammu* **1**, 59.

148. Trivedi JJ (1968) Nagarjun **11**, 503.

149. Deshpande PJ, Pathak SN and Gide JD (1970) In *Advances in Research in Indian Medicine* (eds Udupa KN, Chaturvedi GN and Tripathi,SN), pp. 269-280, Varanasi, Banaras Hindu University.

150. Gupta VS, Prabhakar Rao AVS and Narsimha Rao PL (1963) *Indian J Exp Biol* **1**, 146.

151. Gaind KN, Budhiraja RD and Kaul RN (1966) *Indian J Pharm* **28(9)**, 248.

152. Indap MA, Ambage RY and Gokhle SV (1986) *Indian Drugs* **23(8)**, 447.

153. Ojha D (1967) *Lepr India* **39**, 165.

154. Pandey KP (1967) *Nagarjun* **11**, 91.

155. Upadhyaya YN (1964) *J Med Sci Varanasi* **5**, 97.

156. Inamdar MC, Khurana ML and Rajarama Rao MR (1959) *Indian J Pharm* **21(2)**, 333.

157. Inamdar MC and Rajarama Rao MR (1962) *J Sci Industr Res* **21C**, 345.

158. Gaind KN and Bapna SC (1967) *Indian J Pharm* **29**, 8.

159. Sehgal VN (1967) *Indian J Derm Vener* **33**, 37.

160. Chaudhury RR and Vohora SB (1970) In *Advances of Research of Indian Medicine* (ed Udupa KN, Chaturvedi GN and Tripathi SN), pp. 57-76, Varanasi, Banaras Hindu University.

161. Gupta AS, Singh KP, Maheshwari MM et al (1972) *J Indian Med Prof* **18**, 8256.

162. Gupta SS, Verma SCL Garg VP et al (1967) *Indian J Med Res* **55**, 733.

163. Raghunathan K and Sharma PV (1969) *J Res Indian Med* **4**, 59.

164. Shah DS and Pandya DC (1976) *J Res Indian Med* **11(4)**, 77.

165. Srivastava MR, Gupta SS and Garg VP (1966) *Indian J Physiol Pharmacol* **10**, 12.

166. Sirsi M (1962) *Indian J Pharm* **24**, 83.

167. Shende ST, Balsundaram VR and Sen A (1968) *Indian J Microbiol* **8**, 143.

168. Mahapatra SN (1976) *Indian J Pharm* **38(6)**, 165.

169. Anonymous (1973) *Theories and Philosophies of Medicine*, New Delhi: Department of Philosophy of Medicine and Science, Institute of History of Medicine and Medical Research.

170. Hameed A (1983) Foreward *Medical Elementology* (SB Vohora), New Delhi: Institute of History of Medicine and Medical Research.

171. Iyengar GV, Kollmer WE and Bowen HJM (1978) *The Elemental Composition of Human Tissues and Body Fluids*, Weinheim, New York: Verlag Chemie.

172. Vohora SB (1983) *Medical Elementology*, New Delhi: Institute of History of Medicine and Medical Research.

173. Hameed A and Vohora SB (1990) In: *New Horizons of Health Aspects of Elements* (eds Vohora SB and Dobrowolski JW), pp. 111-202, New Delhi, Jamia Hamdard.

174. Chopra RN, Chopra IC, Handa KL et al (1982) *Chopra's Indigenous Drugs of India*, New Delhi: Academic Publishers.

175. Bhanu KU, Rajadurai S, Sastry KNS et al (1962) *Bull Cent Leather Res Inst*, **8**, 380.

176. Arora RB and Ansari NI (1986) In : *Proceedings Sympo Dermatol & Unani System Med*, HNF Monograph No. 4, pp. 14-28, New Delhi: Hamdard National Foundation.

177. Singh M, Sharma JN, Arora RB et al (1973) *Indian J Pharmacol* **5**, 258.

178. Rao VK, Singh I, Chopra P et al (1986) *Indian J Med Res* **84**, 314.

179. Siddiqui TO (1988) *Times Sci Technol* **7**, 13.

180. Patel RP and Patel KL (1960) *Indian J Pharm* **22(7)**, 174.

181. Trivedi CP, Modi NT, Sarin RR et al (1986) *Indian J Pharmac* **30(3)**, 267.

182. Gupta KC and Chopra IC (1953) *Indian J Med Res* **41**, 459.

183. Budhiraja RD and Garg KN (1973) *Indian J Pharm* **35**, 44.

184. Ghosh D, Anantharaman M and Purushothamaa KK (1980) *Indian J Pharmacol* **12(3)**, 210.

185. Venkatarman S, Vamsadhara C, Nataraja KV et al (1981) *Indian J Physiol Pharmacol* **25**, 102.

186. Satyavati GV, Gupta AK and Tandon N (1987) *Medicinal Plants of India*, vol 2,pp. 72-80, 138-144, 226-229, 272-278, 282-289, 347-351, 354-371, 471-479, 518-530, New Delhi, Indian Council of Medical Research.

187. Mishra SH. Gaud RS, Sharma RA et al (1979) *Indian Drugs* **16**, 141.

188. Tripathi VD, Agarwal SK, Srivastava OP et al (1978) *Indian J Pharmaceut Sci* **40**, 129.

189. Dey BB and Choudhuri MA (1984) *Indian Perfum* **28**, 82.

190. Grover GS and Rao JT (1980) *Perfum u Kosmet* **61(7)**, 256.

191. Gupta KC and Vishwanathan R (1955) *Antibiot Chemother* **5**, 22.

192. Sen K, De G, and Chakraborty R (1983) *Indian J Mycol Res* **21**, 99.

193. Bhat JV and Borker R (1954) *J Sci Industr Res* **13B**, 305.

194. Singh SP, Singh SK and Tripathi SC (1983) *Indian Perfum* **27**, 171.

195. Kishore N, Dube NK, Tripathi RD et al (1982) *Natl Acad Sci Lett* **5(1)**, 9.

196. Roy RG, Madesaya NM, Ghosh RB et al (1976) *Indian J Med Res* **64**, 1451.

197. Sharma SK and Wattal BL (1979) *J Entomol Res* **3(2)**, 172.

198. Chavan SR, Shah MP and Nigam ST (1983) *Bull Haffkine Inst* **11**, 18.

199. Deshmukh PB, Chavan SR and Renapurkar DM (1982) *Pesticides* **16(12)**, 7.

200. Kalyansundaram M and Babu CJ (1982) *Indian J Med Res* **76 (Suppl)**, 102.

201. Malviya BK and Gupta PL (1971) *Indian J Pharm* **33**, 126.

202. Bhargava KP and Singh N (1981) *Indian J Med Res* **73**, 443.

203. Mendiratta PK, Dewan V, Bhatacharya SK et al (1988) *Indian J Med Res* **87(4)**, 384.

204. Dadkar VN, Joshi AG and Jagutse VS (1988) *Indian Drugs* **25(5)**, 172.

205. Balammal R, Thiruvengadam KV, Kamleshwaram L et al (1982) Madurai. *Internal Workshop Pharmacol Biochem Approaches Med Plants*.

206. Das SK (1983) *Antiseptic* **80**, 323.

207. Jalil A (1971) *Asian Med J* **14**, 616.

208. Agarwal SS and Arora RB (1972) *Indian J Pharmacol* **4**, 150.

209. Pillai NGK, Menon RV, Pillai GB et al (1981) *J Res Ayur Siddha* **2(2)**, 122.

210. Ahmad J and Siddiqui TO (1985) In *Development of Unani Drugs from Herbal Sources and the Role of Trace Elements in their Mechanism of Action* (ed. Arora RB), HNF Monograph, p 123, Delhi: Hamdard National Foundation.

211. Dixit SN and Tripathi SC (1975) *Indian Phytopath* **28(1)**, 141.

212. Joglekar GV and Balwani JH (1967) *Maharashtra Med J* **14**, 325.

213. Kato L and Gozsy B (1958) *Arch Int Pharmacodyn* **117**, 52.

214. Srimathi RA and Sreenivasaya M (1963) *Curr Sci* **32(1)**, 11.

215. Turner PN (1964) *Acta Phytother* **11(6)**, 111.

216. Winter AG (1958) *Planta Medica* **6**, 306.

217. Srivastava SC, Khan MSY and Vohora SB (1971) *Indian J Physiol Pharmacol* **15(1)**, 27.

218. *First International Seminar on Unani Medicine* (1987), Abstract Book, pp. 26, 27, 46, 131, New Delhi: Central Council for Research in Unani Medicine and World Health Organization.

219. *Ayurvedic Research Seminar on Skin Diseases*, Abstract Book, pp. 8, 9, 20, 33, 64, Jamnagar: Gujarat Ayurved University.

220. Zafarullah M, Bano H and Vohora SB (1980) *Amer J Chinese Med* **8(4)**, 370.

221. *Symposium on Current Research in Unani Medicine* (1987), New Delhi: Institute of History of Medicine and Medical Research.

222. Vohora SB (1985) *Hamdard Medicus* **28(1)**, 72.

223. Patel RP and Dantwala AS (1958) *Indian J Pharm* **18**, 107.

224. Naryan DS (1969) *Mediscope* **12**, 25.

225. Patel RP and Trivedi BM (1959) *Indian J Med Sci* **13**, 188.

226. Tang W (1992) *Chinese Drugs of Plant Origin*, p. 433, Berlin: Springer Verlag.

227. Khan HA (1996) *Essential and Toxic Elements in Food and Feed Available in Northern India: a model study of Delhi Township* Ph.D. Thesis, New Delhi: Jamia Hamdard.

228. Khan HA (1997) Unpublished data.

229. Khan MSY (1995) Personal communication.

5

Animal Origin Drugs Used in Skin Diseases

5.1 DRUGS OF ANIMAL ORIGIN: A NEGLECTED FIELD OF RESEARCH

Extensive studies are being done in India and elsewhere for research on medicinal plants. There has, however, hardly been any effort to search drugs from animal sources. While bulk of the drugs of Indian materia medica come from Vegetable Kingdom, these systems also use drugs of animal and mineral origin. It is estimated that Ayurveda and Unani-Tibb make use of about 200 drugs of animal origin[1]. Even documentation of claims was not available for motivating the investigators to initiate studies in this area of research. Vohora and Khan[2] from this organisation made a comprehensive survey of Unani literature and documented the claimed utility of these drugs in an illustrated book with classification and therapeutic indices for 32 classes of human ailments including skin diseases.

5.2 UNANI DRUGS OF ZOOLOGICAL ORIGIN WITH CLAIMED UTILITY IN SKIN DISEASES

Tables 5.1 to 5.5 present a list of drugs mentioned in ancient texts of Unani medicine. These drugs are claimed to be useful for the treatment of skin pigmentation, pimples, boils, warts, urticaria, scabies, ring worm, piles, leucoderma, leprosy, malignant ulcers, inflammatory conditions, itching, and insect bites. Their other uses include facilitation of wound healing, improvement of complexion and texture of skin, clearing blemishes, freckles and pock marks and for both depilatory and hair growth promoting effects. The zoological drugs come from animals, birds, snakes, reptiles, insects, flies and amphibious animals. The list includes both whole organisms, and their parts, secretions and excretions. The claims made in Unani texts have not been investigated and offer an almost virgin field to the interested researcher with a dispassionate approach.

Table 5.1 Animal origin drugs attributed with curative effects in skin pigmentation and allied diseases.

S. No.	Scientific name (English name)	Unani name	Remarks
1.	*Bombyx mori* (Silkworm Coccon)	Abresham	Both the worm and its cocoon are used medicinally. The residual cocoon (after the silk thread has been completely removed) contains in its sac, dark brown dried remains of the dead worm. The ash is applied for improving complexion of the skin.
2.	*Hirundu rustica rustica* (Swallow)	Ababil	Blood and excreta are used by application in skin diseases.
3.	*Python reticulatus* (Python)	Azdah	Live animal is burnt and the ash is mixed with honey for external use on piles, leucoderma and skin diseases. Raw flesh is applied on snake bite wounds to absorb toxins.
4.	*Capra hircus* (Goat)	Bakra	Goat's brain is attributed with blood purifying properties. Warm ash of lungs is useful in the treatment of shoe sores. External application of goat urine elicits benificial effect in inflammations and dropsy.
5.	A repltile having long and slender appendages	Bamni	External application of excreta is useful in skin diseases.
6.	N.O. *Anseres* 35 species and sub-species recorded in India (Duck)	Batak	Ash of feathers forms a useful application for freckles and scrofula.
7.	*Coturnix coturnix* (Grey quail)	Bater	Excreta is applied on freckles and lentigo.
8.	*Ploceus philippinensis* (Weaver Bird)	Baya	Excreta forms a useful application for treating moles and skin pigmentation.
9.	*Bos bubalus* (Buffalo)	Bhains	Ash of hooves heals wounds and is good for skin diseases.
10.	*Ovis vignei* (Sheep)	Bhed	External application of bile is useful in skin diseases.
11.	*Pycnotus cofer* (Nightingale)	Bulbul	Excreta is used for the treatment of skin pigmentation.
12.	*Alectoris chukor chukor* (Francolin or Red Partridge)	Chakore	Excreta is applied on skin pigmentation.
13.	N.O. *Chiroptera mega* and micro varieties (large and small bats)	Chamgadar	Excreta is used externally in ring worm.
14.	*Falco biarmicus* (Cherrugh Falcon)	Charzo charagh	Excreta forms a useful application for treating skin diseases.
15.	*Passer domesticus* (Sparrow)	Chidiya	Excreta is applied externally on moles and skin pigmentation.
16.	A kind of fly	Dakori	The files are ground into a paste and applied externally for the treatment of skin pigmentation.
17.	*Streptopelia chinensis* (Spotted Dove)	Fakhta	Excreta is mixed with vinegar and applied in cases of skin pigmentation.

(Contd.)

S. No.	Scientific name (English name)	Unani name	Remarks
18.	*Bos taurus* (Cow)	Gai	Milk and curd improve complexion. Cow milk facilitates healing of wounds, External application of urine cures skin pigmentation.
19.	*Canis aureus* (Jackal)	Geedar	Excreta is applied externally for treating skin diseases.
20.	Family: *Perameliadoe* many species (Bandicoot)	Ghoonse	Blood cures warts and scars.
21.	*Equs caballus* (Horse)	Ghora	Blood is applied on boils and urine on ring worm.
22.	*Pseudogyps bengalensis* (Vulture)	Gidh	Excreta is used externally in cases of skin pigmentation.
23.	*Varanus bengalensis* *Varanus salvator* (Monitor)	Goh	Ash of flesh is useful in cutaneous disorders.
24.	A bird resembling Falcon but smaller than it	Jarra	Local application of excreta is used in cases of skin pigmentation.
25.	*Calamba livia* (Blue Rock Pigeon)	Kabootar	Eggs improve complexion of the skin.
26.	*Oryctolagus cuniculus* (Rabbit)	Khargosh	External application of blood on scalp promotes hair growth.
27.	*Eudynamis scalopaeus malyana* (Cuckoo)	Koyal	Flesh, when taken orally, improves complexion of skin and prevents premature greying of hair.
28.	*Hyaena hyaena hyaena* (Hyena)	Lakarbagga	Oral intake of flesh prevents bilious humours and improves complexion.
29.	*Ciconia ciconia* (White Stork)	Laklak	External application of blood and excreta is useful in skin diseases.
30.	*Centropus sinensis sinensis* (Crow Pheasant or Coucol)	Laklak	External application of blood and excreta is useful in skin diseases.
31.	*Pavo cristatus* (Peacock)	Mor	Blood, mixed with other medicaments, forms a useful application for malignant skin ulcers. Ash of bones is applied in cases of leucoderma and skin pigmentation.
32.	*Nyroca ferina* (Pochard)	Murghabi	External application of brain paste is useful in inflammatory conditions and exfoliation of skin.
33.	*Gallus domesticus* (Fowl)	Murgh	Intake of flesh improves complexion. Egg albumin is astringent and it is used for healing of wounds and burns. The oil extracted from egg yolk is used as an inunction for growth of the hair of beard and moustaches and as an embrocation for maturing abscesses. Eggs are mixed with honey and vinegar to form a useful application for clearing blemishes and freckles of face and for relief in inflammatory conditions. Egg shell powder is used in urticaria, skin diseases and for healing wounds.
34.	*Coracas benghalensis* (Roller or Blue Jay)	Nilkanth	External application of excreta is useful in cases of skin pigmentation.

(Contd.)

S. No.	Scientific name (English name)	Unani name	Remarks
35.	*Camelus dromedarius* (Camel)	Oont	Ash of flesh is used externally in urticaria and other skin diseases. Milk is attributed with antiinflammatory properties and curd is Claimed to be of value of leprosy.
36.	A bird found near water	Poi	Bile is useful in skin pigmentation.
37.	Class: *Reptilia* N.O. : *Ophidia* Many species (Snake)	Saanp	The snake is eviscerated, stuffed with some medicinal leaves and sutured. It is then put in hot ash. After it has been well cooked, the sutures are opened, the leaves are taken out and pulverized. This powder is claimed to cure leucoderma within 24 hours of application. Ash of black snakes is applied with olive oil for the treatment of scrofula and with vinegar in alopecia. Oil extracted from snakes and snake slough is incorporated in ointments for use in leucoderma. Bile is boiled with oil to form a useful application for moles and leprosy.
38.	*Os sepiae* : internal shell of *Sepia officinalis* (Sea foam or Cuttle fish bones)	Samundarphen	External application of the powdered foam is good for treating inflammations, skin pigmentation and irritating skin diseases e.g. ringworm, scabies and insect bites. It brings about relief by causing local sedation in these cases.
39.	*Ostrea edulis* (Oyster shell)	Seep	Pulverized shells possess hemostatic, vaso constrictor and astringent properties. The powder is useful in burns and facial marks.
40.	*Hystrix indica* (Indian Porcupine)	Sehi	Fat is used as local application to cure skin pigmentation.
41.	*Mel* (Honey) produced by several bees e.g. *Apis mellifera, Apis dorsata, Apis indica* etc.	Shehad	It improves skin complexion. Application with vinegar and salt is useful in skin pigmentation, inflammatory conditions and leprosy.
42.	*Sturthio camelus* (Ostrich)	Shutarmurgh	Excreta is applied to clear pock marks and skin pigmentation.
43.	*Panthera pardus* (Leopard)	Tendua	Blood forms a good external application for use in cases of skin pigmentation.
44.	*Locusta migratoria* (Locust)	Tiddi	Appendages are ground and mixed with vinegar for application on scabies, moles and skin pigmentation.
45.	*Pieris napi* (Butterfly)	Titari	Paste of whole organism with vinegar is used externally in moles, scabies, skin pigmentation and leprosy.
46.	*Peritacula krameri borealis* (Parrot)	Tota	Intake of flesh facilitates healing of wounds and is useful in skin pigmentation. Excreta is applied externally in skin pigmentation.

Table 5.2.   Animal origin drugs used in alopecia and baldness

S. No.	Scientific Name (English Name)	Unani Name	Part*
1.	*Daboia russel vel elegans and Echis carinata* varieties commonly occur in India (Viper)	Aphai	Flesh (Oral use)
2.	Hair	Bal	Oil extracted from human hairs
3.	*Ovis vignei* (Sheep)	Bhed	Ash of bones
4.	*Canis lupus* (Wolf)	Bhediya	Fat
5.	Class : *Archnida* N.O. : *Scorpiones* Many species (Scorpion)	Bichoo	Ash of whole organism
6.	*Gecko vertillatus* or *Hemidactylus flavivirdis* (House Lizard)	Chhipkali	Dried liver mixed with olive oil.
7.	*Mus rattus* (Rat)	Chooha	Excreta with vinegar and honey
8.	*Equs asinus* (Donkey or Ass)	Gadha	Ash of penis mixed with olive oil
9.	Family : *Perameladiae* Many species (Bandicoot)	Ghoonse	Excreta with honey
10.	*Chameleon vulgaris Chameleon zeylanicus* (Chameleon or Garden hizard)	Girgit	Fat
11.	*Equs burchelli* (Zebra)	Gorkhar	Dried pulverized lungs with honey and gum tragacanth
12.	*Elephus maximus* (Elephant)	Haathi	Ash or fine powder of teeth (Ivory)
13.	*Cervus axis* (Deer)	Haran	Fat
14.	*Dicrurus macrocercus* (Black Drongo)	Jhanpul	Whole bird (alongwith a large black bee) is boiled in seasame oil.
15.	*Corvus splendens splendens* (Crow)	Kaua	Whole live bird is kept in a utensil alongwith some iron dust and vinegar. The utensil is then buried in horse dung for 40 days. This procedure causes disintegration of the bird's flesh and an oily substance is exuded. This is useful for blackening hair and stimulating hair growth.
16.	Hybrid offspring of a male ass (*Equs assinus*) and a mare (*Equs cabbalus*) (Mule)	Khachar	Hoof rubbed in oil
17.	*Cimex lectularius Cimex rotundatus* (Bed bug)	Khatmal	Paste of bugs
18.	*Pedicula asiatica* (Jungle Bush Quail)	Lawa	Ash of bones with olive oil.

(Contd.)

S. No.	Scientific name (English name)	Unani name	Part*
19.	*Musca domestica* (House Fly)	Makkhi	100 flies put in seasame oil for 40 days and then filtered; filtrate is used.
20.	*Melursus ursinus* (Bear)	Reechh	Fat
21.	Class : *Reptilia* N.O.: *Ophidia* Many species (Snake)	Saanp	Snake casting in olive oil
22.	*Sacchobranchus fossilies* (Singi Fish)	Singi Macchli	Ash of fish
23.	*Sus scrofa* (Wild Boar)	Suar	Bile with honey and black pepper
24.	N.O. : *Cleoptera* Family : *Meloidae* 11 genera of which 3 are important viz.: *Canthrasis, Mylabris* and *Melae* (Blister Bee or Cantharides)	Telni Makkhi	*Cantharidine*: a fatty acid contained in dried insects is incorporated in hair oils and pomades.

*All medicaments used externally except Viper flesh which is given orally.

Table 5.3 Animal origin drugs locally applied as depilatory agents.

S. No.	Scientific Name (English Name)	Unani Name	Part used
1.	*Macaca mulatta* (Monkey)	Bandar	Blood
2.	N.O. : *Chiroptera Mega* and *micro* varieties (Big and small bats)	Chamgadar	Blood
3.	A kind of fly	Dakori	Paste made of ground flies
4.	*Chameleon vulgaris Chameleon zeylanicus* (Chameleon or Garden Lizard)	Girgit	Blood

Table 5.4. Animal origin drugs used in piles

S.No.	Scientific Name (English Name)	Unani Name	Remarks
1.	*Python retinculatus* (Python)	Azdah	Ash is mixed with honey and locally applied.
2.	A kind of sea shell	Azfarulteeb	Powder is used externally
3.	*Ardea cinerea* (Heron)	Bagula	External application of fat
4.	*Bos taurus* (Ox)	Bail	External application of fat
5.	*Capra hircus* (Goat)	Bakra	Freshly removed hide is applied on piles
6.	*Macaca mulatta* (Monkey)	Bandar	External application of flesh
7.	*Cervus duvacuceli* (Antelope or Stag)	Baraseenga	Powder or ash of horns is dusted on piles.
8.	*Francolinus pondicerious* (A bird resembling Partridge)	Bharraka	External application of flesh
9.	*Ovis vignei* (Sheep)	Bhed	Curd and urine are used topically.
10.	*Canis lupus* (Wolf)	Bhediya	External application of ash of tibial bone or penis.
11.	Family : *Feledoe* many species (Cat)	Billi	External application of flesh
12.	*Milvus migrans* (Pariah kite)	Cheel	Long term ingestion of flesh with some herbal preparations.
13.	*Mus rattus* (Rat)	Chooha	External application of flesh
14.	Common species: *Caprotermes ceylonicus* *Captotermes heimal* *Heterostesmes indicola* (White ant or Termite)	Deemak	Whole organism is made into a paste with fat from Ox hump and applied locally.
15.	*Bos taurus* (Cow)	Gai	External application of excreta with vinegar.
16.	*Rhinoceros unicornis* (Rhinoceros)	Gainda	Fumigation from burnt horns and hooves is useful in piles.
17.	*Pila globosa* (Apple snail)	Ghonga	Intake of calx (*Kushta*) of whole organism.
18.	Family : *Peramelidoe* many species (Bandicoot)	Ghoonse	Fumigation from burnt skin.
19.	N.O. : *Coleoptera* many species from 9 families (Beetle)	Gobrilla	External application of a paste prepared from whole organisms.
20.	*Elephus maximus* (Elephant)	Haathi	External application of fine powder or ash of skin with wax.

(Contd.)

S. No.	Scientific name (English name)	Unani name	Remarks
21.	*Hirundo medicinalis* (Leech)	Jonk	Local application of dried powder with olive oil and vinegar.
22.	Family : *Eleterdae* Genus : *Pyrophyrus* many species (Fire fly or Glow worm)	Jugnu	Local application of dried pulverized organisms with egg albumin.
23.	*Testudo elegans* (Tortoise)	Kachhua	Fumigation from burnt bones.
24.	*Corvus splendens splendens* (Crow)	Kaua	External application of dried blood
25.	*Scilla serrata* (Crab)	Kekra/Sartan	External application of ash.
26.	*Oryctolagus cuniculus* (Rabbit)	Khargosh	External application of skin.
27.	*Pheritima posthuma* (Earthworms)	Kharateen	Worms are made into a paste for local application.
28.	*Canis familiaris* (Dog)	Kutta	Ash of bones is used as a dusting powder.
29.	*Viverricula indica* (Civet Cat)	Mashak Bilai	External application of civet: an odourless secretion contained in a pouch situated between anus and genital organs of civet cat.
30.	*Rana tigriana* (Frog)	Mendak	Decoction is used for topical application
31.	*Cera* (Wax)	Mome	External application.
32.	*Corallium rubrum* (Coral)	Moonga	External application of powder.
33.	*Pavo cristatus* (Peacock)	Mor	External application of excreta.
34.	*Pincatada* (Pearls)	Moti	Powder or ash are used for local application.
35.	*Herpestis edwardsii* *Herpestis mungo* (Mongoose)	Nevla	Blood is boiled in olive oil and filtered, the filtrate is used.
36.	*Camelus dromedarius* (Camel)	Oont	Milk and fat are used for topical application.
37.	A bird found near water	Poi	External application of flesh.
38.	Class : *Reptilia* N.O. : *Ophidia* many species (Snake)	Saanp	Fumigation from snake castings.
39.	*Grus antigone antigone* (Indian Crane)	Saras	External application of flesh.
40.	*Sus scrofa* (Wild Boar)	Suar	External application of bile.
41.	*Locusta migratoria* (Locust)	Tiddi	Fumigation from burnt locusts.
42.	*Strunus vulgaris* (Starling)	Tiliyar	External application of flesh.

Table 5.5. Animal origin drugs used for healing burns and wounds

(A) ORAL USE

S. No.	Scientific Name (English Name)	Unani Name	Part Used
1.	*Bos taurus* (Ox)	Bail	Beef soup
2.	*Bos bubalus* (Buffalo)	Bhains	Meat extract
3.	*Pisces* (Fish)	Machhli	Isinglass, eggs and oil from liver
4.	*Corallium rubrum* (Coral)	Moonga	Powder

(B) EXTERNAL USE

S. No.	Scientific Name (English Name)	Unani Name	Part Used
1.	*Spongia officinalis* (Sponge)	Aspanj	Powder or small pieces.
2.	*Bos taurus* (Ox/Cow)	Bail/Gai	Excreta, ash of horns and hooves.
3.	*Capra hircus* (Goat)	Bakra	Spinal cord, blood exuded from spleen, powder of horns and sebacious secretion (*Zoophyatar*)
4.	*Macaca mulatta* (Monkey)	Bandar	Ash of flesh.
5.	*Cervus duvacuceli* (Antellope or Stag)	Baraseenga	Ash of horns.
6.	*Bos bubalus* (Buffalo)	Bhains	Ash of hooves and horns
7.	*Ovis vignei* (Sheep)	Bhed	Blood, excreta and sebacious secretion (*Zoophyatar*)
8.	*Pycnotus cafer* (Nightingale)	Bulbul	Ash of feathers.
9.	*Axis axis* (Speckled Deer)	Cheetal	Ash of hooves.
10.	*Leptoptilos dubius* (Adjutant Stork)	Dheenk	Dried pulverized skin
11.	*Rhinoceros unicornis* (Rhinoceros)	Gainda	Fat with seasame oil.
12.	*Pila globosa* (Apple Snail)	Ghonga	Ash of Whole organism.
13.	*Pseudogyps bengalensis* (Vulture)	Gidh	Ash of feathers

(Contd.)

S. No.	Scientific name (English name)	Unani name	Part Used
14.	*Elephus maximus* (Elephant)	Haathi	i. Ash of skin ii. Powered Ivory
15.	*Cervus axis* (Deer)	Haran	Ash of horns
16.	*Calumba livia* (Blue Rock Pigeon)	Kabootar	Excreta
17.	*Scilla serrata* (Crab)	Kekra/Sartan	Ash of whole organism
18.	*Treron sphenura sphenura* (Wedge tailed Green Pigeon)	Kokla	Ash of feathers.
19.	*Pheretima posthuma* (Earth Worms)	Kharateen	Dried pulverized worms
20.	*Vulpes bengalensis* (Fox)	Lomri	Ash of skin
21.	*Acridothores tristis tristis* (Common Myna)	Maina	Ash of flesh
22.	*Aranca diodema* (Spider)	Makri	White spider web
23.	*Rana tigriana* (Frog)	Mendak	Flesh and brain
24.	*Cera* (Wax)	Mome	Used as vehicle for ointments
25.	*Corallium rubrum* (Coral)	Moonga	Powder
26.	*Gallus domesticus* (Fowl)	Murgh	Egg albumin, egg shell powder
27.	*Boselaphus tragocamelus* (Blue Bull)	Nil Gai	Ash of horns
28.	*Camelus dromedarius* (Camel)	Oont	Ash of hairs
29.	*Mustella zibellina* (Sable)	Samur	Ash of hairs
30.	*Ostrea edulis* (Oyester shell)	Seep	Powder
31.	*Panthera pardus* (Leopard)	Tendua	Flesh and fat cooked with water and olive oil.
32.	*Perittacula krumeri borealis* (Parrot)	Tota	Flesh
33.	*Lutra lutra* (Common Otter)	Ud Bilao	Ash of tongue
34.	*Balaena* (Whale)	Whale	Fat

5.3 REFERENCES

1. Puri HS (1970) *Nagarjun* **13**, 21.

2. Vohora SB and Khan MSY (1978) *Animal Origin Drugs Used in Unani Medicine,* ed 1, pp. 84, 85, New Delhi: Vikas Publishing House and Institute of History of Medicine and Medical Research.

6

Leucoderma

6.1 LEUCODERMA: A CHALLENGE TO MEDICAL SCIENCE

Leucoderma, an idiopathic patchy depigmentation of skin, is a challenge to medical science. The chronic form of disease is very stubborn, resistant to therapy and causes immense misery to the patients. They are not socially accepted, remain dejected, disturbed and develop inferiority complex. The etiology of the disease is not precisely known and so it is attributed to a variety of causative factors. These include nutritional, metabolic, hereditary, neurogenic and autoimmune disorders, protozoal infestation, stress etc.[1,2]

The most accepted theory is that the disease is due to defect in the metabolism of tyrosine which fails to be converted into Melanin. Figure 6.1 depicts the various steps involved in the metabolic pathways of this amino acid. The factors involved in these reactions include optimum skin pH (5.6 to 6.8), ultra violet light, tyrosinase (a copper containing enzyme), diphosphatide pyridine nucleotide (DPN), nicotic, pentothinic and ascorbic acids, and melanophore stimulating enzyme. Of the various factors enumerated, tyrosinase is of principal importance. Melanin (a polymeric black pigment present in skin and hair) is formed in granules called melanosomes that are rich in tyrosinase. Tyrosine must be activated in human skin to enable it to catalyse the oxidation of tyrosine to melanin. This is fascilatated by ultra violet light. The activity of this enzyme is inhibited by copper deficiency. SH-group forming covalent bonds with copper (possibly by lack of UV light), melatonin (a substance secreted at nerve endings), and tryptophan pyrrolase (an enzyme causing excretion of indole in the urine of leucoderma patients).

The disease has also been reported to result from the presence of an unidentified neurohormone that can lighten the melanocytes[2,3]. Because of the poor understanding about its etiology and pathogenesis, not much headway could be made towards development of effective therapeutic agents for the disease. The search should, therefore, continue.

6.2 AYURVEDIC AND UNANI CONCEPTS

According to Ayurvedic medicine the skin is composed of seven layers: *Abavabani, Lohita, Sweta, Tambra, Vedini, Rohini* and *Manasdhara*. The pigment granules (*Bhrajka pittya* or melanin) are contained in *Jambra* and *Vedini* layers of the skin. *Switra* (leucoderma) has

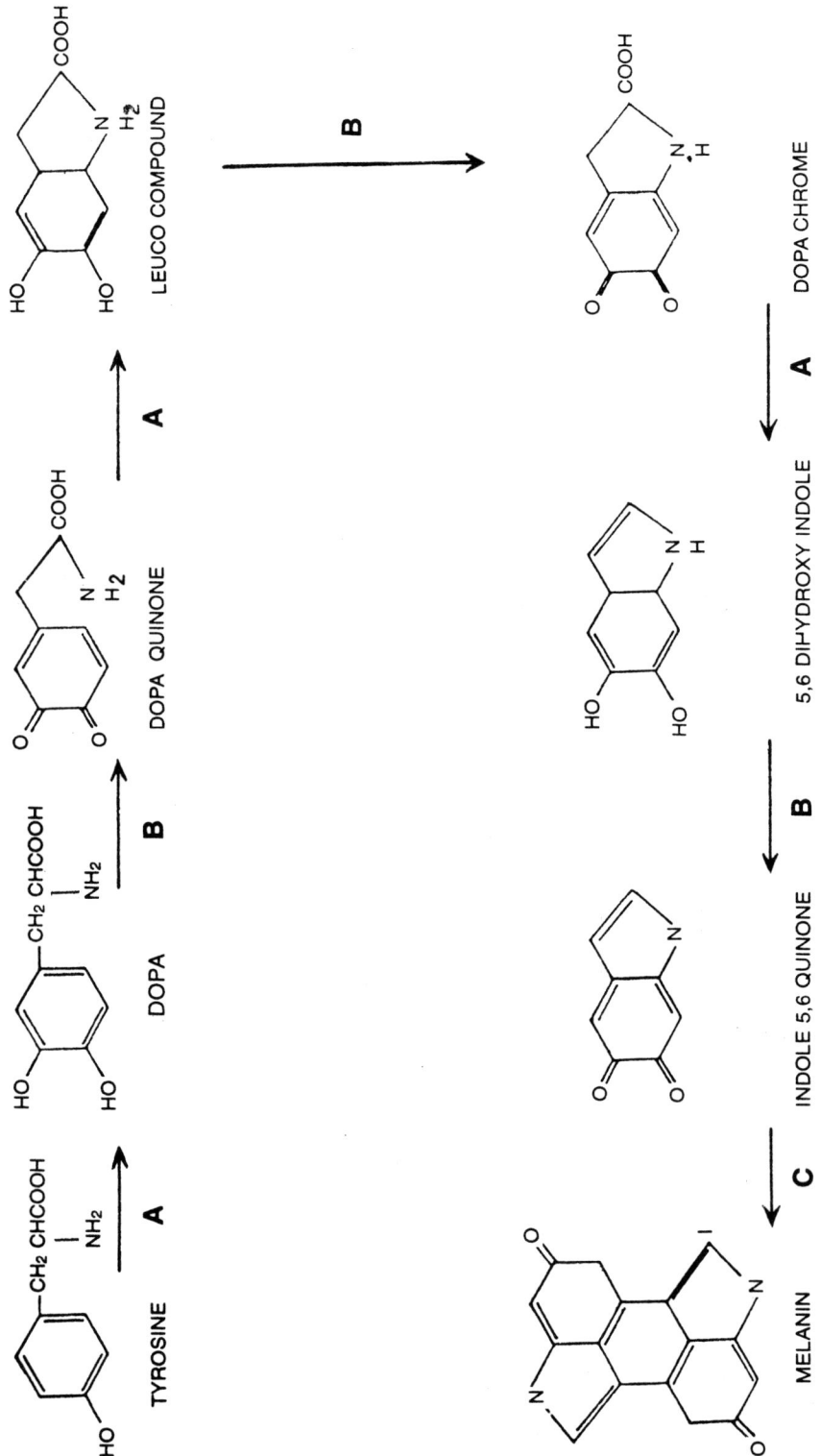

Fig. 6.1 Metabolic Pathways in Synthesis of Melanin from Tyrosine

A : HYDROXYLATION
B : OXIDATION
C : POLYMERIZATION

been described in Ayurvedic texts as a kind of localised *Kusta* (leprosy) and is attributed to the vitiation of *Rasa* (plasma), *Mansa* (muscle tissue) and *Medha dhatus* (adipose tissue). The disease is non-exudative in nature but is associated with itching and hypersensitiveness in majority of the cases. The prognosis is good and the disease is curable if the patches are fresh, few, not connected with each other, not associated with burns and if the hair over these patches have not turned white[4,5].

Bars-Abyaz (Vitiligo) according to Unani-Tibb may be due to: a) excessive coldness or moisture in the *Mizaj* (temperament) of the body as a whole or in a particular part, b) excessive *Balgham-e-Kham* (raw phelgm) in blood, c) weakness in particular part of the skin reducing its capacity to utilize the nutrients absorbed from the blood and convert them into normal pigments, d) excessive use of *Ghiza-e-Ghaliz* (foods which take more time for digestion and absorption), and e) excessive use of *Ghiza-e-Barid* (cold foods like milk, yoghurt etc). According to Avicenna (1037 AD) the causative substance producing the disease is much concentrated and adherent to the structures and is not transformed according to the requirement of normal colour. He further adds that the energy for expelling it out is also inadequate causing obstruction in the metabolism[2]. It is interesting to note that his concept regarding the etiology of the disease (stated in different terminology) is not very much different from what is known today.

The treatment is done by using herbomineral products in both the systems.

6.3 MEDICINAL PLANTS USED FOR THE TREATMENT OF LEUCODERMA

A large number of medicinal plants have been described in folklore, Indian medicinal systems (Ayurveda, Unani-Tibb, Siddha medicine), homoeopathy, and modern medicine as useful in leucoderma (Table 6.1). These are used both as simples and in compound formulations by oral route and also by topical applications[2,4-10].

Table 6.1 Medicinal plants used in leucoderma[4-10]

1.	*Abrus precatorius* LInn	2.	*Acacia catechu* Willd
3.	*Acacia foprnesiana* Willd	4.	*Acacia ferruginea* DC
5.	*Acacia nilotica* Del	6.	*Aconitum chasmanthum* Stapf
7.	*Aconitum falconeri* Stapf	8.	*Aconitum rugata* Lam
9.	*Acorus calamus* Linn	10.	*Adhatoda vasica* Nees
11.	*Aglaia odoratissima* Blume	12.	*Albizia amara* Boivin
13.	*Albizia lebbek* Benth	14.	*Allium cepa* Linn
15.	*Allium sativum* Linn	16.	*Alpinea galanga* Willd
17.	*Alpinia khulanjan* Sheriff	18.	*Alpinia officinarum* Hance
19.	*Alstonia scholaris* R Br	20.	*Altingea excelasa* Noronha
21.	*Amararanthus tristis* Linn	22.	*Ammi majus* Linn
23.	*Anacardium occidentale* Linn	24.	*Anacyclus pyrethrum* DC
25.	*Amemone obustifolia* D Don	26.	*Anethum sowa* Roxb
27.	*Anthriscus cerifolium* Hoffm	28.	*Apium graveolens* Linn
29.	*Aquillaria agallocha* Roxb	30.	*Argemone mexicana* Linn
31.	*Aristolchia indica* Linn	32.	*Artemisia siversiana* Willd

(Contd.)

33. *Astragalus hamosus* Linn
34. *Atropa belladonna* Linn
35. *Azadirachta indica* A juss
36. *Bacopa monnieri* Linn
37. *Balanites aegyptica* Del
38. *Baleospermum montanum* Muell-Arg
39. *Bambusa arundinaeca* Willd
40. *Barleria priontis* Linn
41. *Barleria strigosa* Willd
42. *Bauhinea variegata* Linn.
43. *Blepharis edulis* Pers
44. *Boswelia serrata* Roxb
45. *Brassica campestris* Linn
46. *Brassica nigra* Koch
47. *Butea monosperma* (Lam) Kuntz
48. *Calamus rotang* Linn
49. *Calotropis gigantea* R Br
50. *Canscora decussata* Roem et Sch.
51. *Capparis sepiaria* Linn
52. *Careya arborea* Roxb
53. *Carthamus tinctorius* Linn
54. *Carum carvi* Linn
55. *Casearia esculenta* Roxb
56. *Cassia absus* Linn
57. *Cassia angustifolia* Vahl
58. *Cassia tora* Linn
59. *Cedrus deodara* (Roxb) Lour
60. *Celastrus paniculata* Willd
61. *Centella asiatica* Urban
62. *Centipeda minima* Br et Asch
63. *Centratherum anthelminitcum* Kuntz
64. *Cephalandra indica* Naud
65. *Chenopodium album* Linn
66. *Cinnamomum zeylanicum* Blume
67. *Cissus adanta* Roxb
68. *Cissus setosa* Roxb
69. *Citrullus colocynthis* Schrad
70. *Cleome brachycarpa* Vahl
71. *Cleome chelidonni* Linn
72. *Cleome icosandra* Linn
73. *Clerodendron infortunatum* Linn
74. *Clitorea ternatea* Linn
75. *Commiphora agalocha* Engl
76. *Commiphora mukul* Hook ex Stocks
77. *Convolvulus scammonia* Linn
78. *Coptis teeta* Wall
79. *Coriandrum sativum* Linn
80. *Corydalis govniana* Wall
81. *Croton tiglium* Linn
82. *Cuminum cyminum* Linn
83. *Curcuma angustifolia* Roxb
84. *Curcuma aromatica* Salisb
85. *Curcuma caesia* Roxb
86. *Curcuma longa* Linn
87. *Curcuma zedoaria* Rosc
88. *Dalbergia sissoo* Roxb
89. *Datura metel* Linn
90. *Datura stramonium* Linn
91. *Delphinium denudatum* Wall
92. *Dioscorea bulbifera* Linn
93. *Dolichos biflorus* Linn
94. *Dolichos falcatus* Klun
95. *Drogea volubilis* Benth
96. *Ecballium elatarium* A Rich
97. *Eclipta alba* Massk
98. *Eclipta erecta* Lamk
99. *Embelia ribes* Burm f
100. *Emblica officinalis* Gaertn
101. *Enhydra fluctuans* Lour
102. *Eruca sativa* Mill
103. *Euphorbia neriifolia* Linn
104. *Evolvulus alsinoides* Linn
105. *Fagonia cretica* Linn
106. *Feronia limonia* Swingl
107. *Ficus carica* Linn
108. *Ficus hispida* Linn
109. *Ficus microcarpa* E Vill
110. *Ficus racemosa* Linn
111. *Ficus religiosa* Linn
112. *Ficus tsiela* Roxb
113. *Fumaria indica* Pugsley
114. *Geranium wallichianum* Sweet
115. *Girardinia heteraphylla* DC
116. *Gisekia pharnaceoides* Linn

(Contd.)

117. *Glorisa superba* Linn.
118. *Gymnema sylevestre* R Br
119. *Gynocardia odorata* R Br
120. *Hemidesmus indicus* R Br
121. *Heracleum candicans* Wall
122. *Heracleum canescens* Lindl
123. *Heracleum pinnatum* Wild
124. *Holarrhena antidysentrica* Wall
125. *Holostemma annulare* K Schum
126. *Hydnocarpus kurzii* Warb
127. *Hyoscymus niger* Linn
128. *Indigofera tinctoria* Linn
129. *Ipomea hederacea* Jacq
130. *Ipomea reninformis* Choisy
131. *Ipomea raptans* Poir
132. *Iris versicolor* Linn
133. *Lactuca scariola* Linn
134. *Lamprachenium microcephalum* Benth
135. *Lawsonia inermis* Linn
136. *Lepidium sativum* Linn
137. *Lolium femulentum* Linn
138. *Luffa acutangula* Roxb
139. *Lupinus albus* Linn
140. *Macrotomea benthame* DC
141. *Macrotomea perennis* Bois
142. *Martynia annua* Linn
143. *Melia azardirach* Bois
144. *Melia azadirachta* Linn
145. *Meliotus alba* Desr
146. *Meliotus officinalis* Desr
147. *Mentha sylvestris* Linn
148. *Mimosa pudica* Linn
149. *Moringa concanensis* Nimmo
150. *Moringa oleifera* Lam
151. *Murraya koenigii* Spreng
152. *Musa paradisiaca* Linn
153. *Mussaenda glabrata* Hutich
154. *Nardostachys jatamansi* DC
155. *Nelumbo mucifera* Gaertn
156. *Nerium odorum* Soland
157. *Nicotiana rustica* Linn
158. *Nicotiana tabacum* Linn
159. *Nigella sativa* Linn
160. *Nymphaea stellata* Willd
161. *Ocimum basilicum* Linn
162. *Ocimum sanctum* Linn
163. *Onosma bracteatum* Wall
164. *Onosma echioides* Linn
165. *Operculiana turpethum* Silva Manso
166. *Opuntia dillunii* Haw
167. *Origanum majorana* Linn
168. *Oroxylon indicum* Vent
169. *Orthosiphon pallidus* Royle
170. *Ougeinia oojeinensis* Hochr
171. *Oxystelma esculenta* R Br
172. *Paederia foetida* Linn
173. *Pandanus tectorius* Sol
174. *Paris polyphylla* Smith
175. *Pentatropis cynachoides* R Br
176. *Phaseolus radiatus* Lour
177. *Picrorrhiza kurroa* Royle ex Benth
178. *Pinus sylvestris* Linn
179. *Piper longum* Linn
180. *Plantanus orientalis* Linn
181. *Plumbago indica* Linn
182. *Plumbago zeylanica* Linn
183. *Pongamia pinnata* Merr
184. *Prospis juliflora* DC
185. *Prunus amygdalus* Stok
186. *Prunus cerasoidea* D Don
187. *Prunus perrica* Batsch
188. *Psoralea corylifolia* Linn
189. *Pterocarpus marsupium* Roxb
190. *Punica granatum* Linn
191. *Randia dumetorum* Lam
192. *Ranunculus scleratus* Linn
193. *Raphanus sativus* Linn
194. *Rheum emodi* Wall
195. *Ricinus communis* Linn
196. *Rubia cordifolia* Linn
197. *Rumex vesicarium* Linn
198. *Sapindus mukorossi* Gaertn
199. *Sasbania sesban* Merr
200. *Saussurea lappa* Clarke
201. *Semecarpus anacardium* Linn
202. *Solanum indicum* Linn

(Contd.)

203. *Solanum melongena* Linn	204. *Solanum nigrum* Linn
205. *Sphaeranthus indicus* Linn	206. *Spinacea oleracea* Linn
207. *Strychnos nux vomica* Linn	208. *Swertia chirata* Buch Ham
209. *Tamarix articulata* Vahl	210. *Tamarix indica* Linn
211. *Tamarix troupii* Hole	212. *Tecomelia undulata* Seem
213. *Tectona grandis* Linn	214. *Terminalia arjuna* Wright & Arn
215. *Terminalia belerica* Roxb	216. *Terminalia chebula* Retz
217. *Terminalia citrina* Roxb	218. *Thevetia neriifolia* Juss
219. *Tricholepis glaberrima* DC	220. *Trichosanthes cucurmeriana* Linn
221. *Trigonella foenum graecum* Linn	222. *Urginea indica* Kunth
223. *Urtica dioica* Linn	224. *Uritica parviflora* Roxb
225. *Vicia faba* Linn	226. *Viola serpens* Wall
227. *Viola triculor* Linn	228. *Vilex negundo* Linn
229. *Vitex trifolia* Linn	230. *Wedelia calendulacea* Less
231. *Widhania somnifera* Dunal	232. *Wrightia tinctoria* R Br
233. *Xanthium strumarium* Linn	234. *Zanthoxylum acanthopodium* DC
235. *Zanthoxylum alatum* Roxb	236. *Zanthoxylum oxyphyllum* Edgew
237. *Zingiber officinale* Rosc	

6.4 SCIENTIFIC INVESTIGATIONS

Very few plants from the vast number listed in the previous section have been subjected to scientific (experimental and clinical) investigation. Prominent among these are *Ammi majus* and *Psoralea corylifolia* which have been extensively studied for pharmacognositc, chemical, pharmacological, toxicological, clinical and cultivation aspects. *Ammi majus* was specifically used in vitiligo by Arab physicians. This plant was not available in India. Therefore the Unani practitioners here adopted the seeds of *Psoralea corylifolia* for use in this diseases. Cultivation of *Ammi majus* was later taken up at various places in the country including Jammu, Hyderabad, Lucknow, and New Delhi. Cutivation was also done at the drug farm of Institute of History of Medicine and Medical Research, New Delhi (merged with Jamia Hamdard in 1989). Drugs from these two plants are used not only in traditional medicine but also in modern medicine. These plants are, therefore, described in details.

6.4.1 *Ammi majus* Linn

History and Chemistry

The plant is called *Aatrilal* in Unani medicine as it resembles leg of a bird. The oldest record of its use in vitiligo dates back to eleventh century AD. This is mentioned in a review by Ibn Beitar[2]. The fruits and seeds of the plant have been extensively investigated for chemical components[11-13]. Details of such studies are omitted for the sake of brevity. The active principles are furocoumaris: ammoidin (8 methoxypsoralen or xanthotoxin), ammidin (8 ammylenoxy psoralen or imperatonin), majudin (5 methoxy psoralen or bergapten), isopimpinellin, marmesin, marmesinin, ammajine, isoimperotinin, alloimperaotnin etc. These are shown in Figure 6.2.

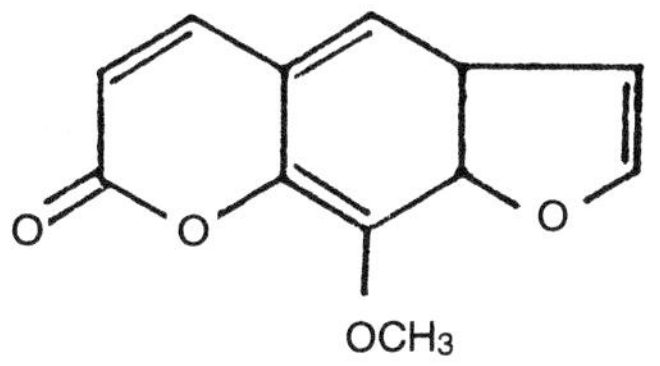

AMMODIN
OR
8 - METHOXY PSORALEN
OR
XANTHOTOXIN

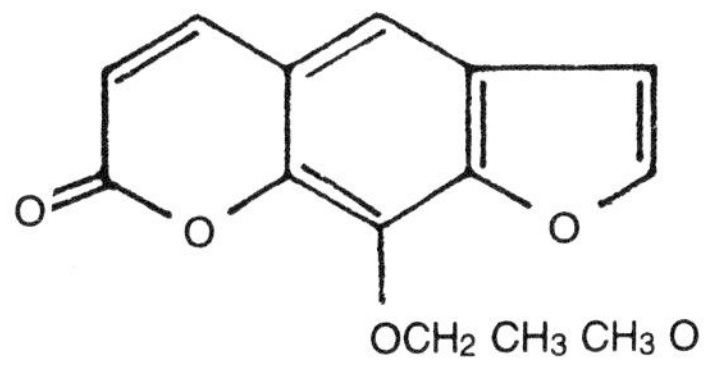

AMMIDIN
OR
8 - AMMYLENOXY PSORALEN
OR
IMPEROTONIN

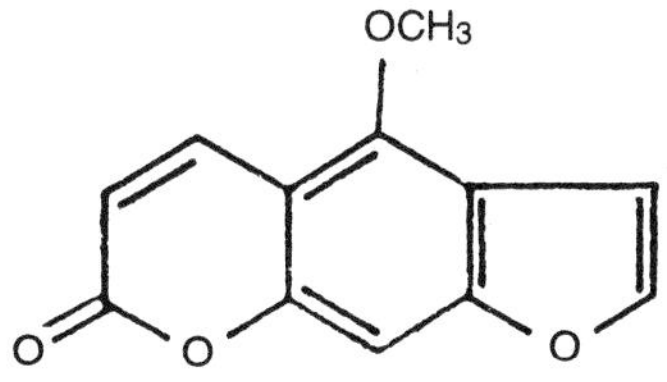

MAJUDIN
OR
5 METHOXY PSORALEN
OR
BERGAPTEN

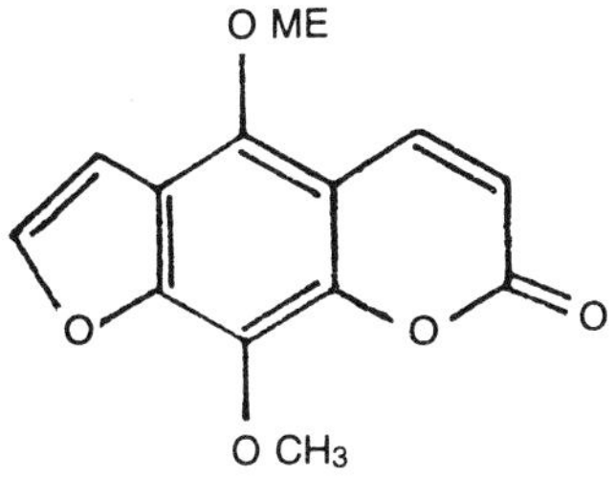

ISOIMPINELLIN

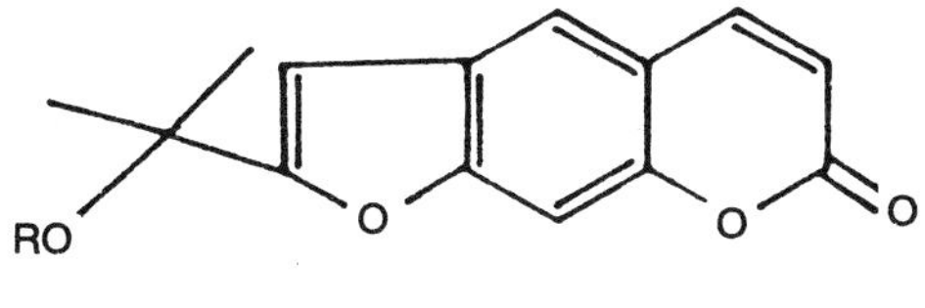

MARMESIN
R = H
MARMESININ
R = Glu

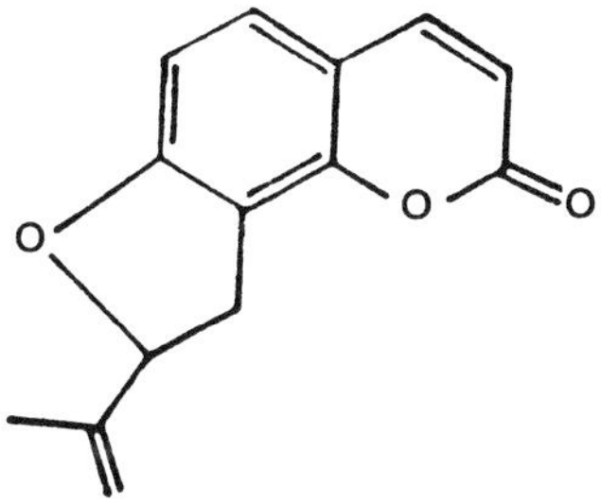

MAJURIN

Fig. 6.2 SOME CHEMICAL PRINCIPLES ISOLATED FROM *Ammi majus* LINN

Efficacy in Leucoderma

The clinical efficacy of the drug has been proved beyond doubt as numerous reports are available on this aspect[14-18]. If, however, the disease is associated with destruction of melanocytes, the drug is ineffective. A perusal of the various clinical trial reports showed that the crude drug (powder of fruits and seeds) was used in the dose range of 20-75 mg/kg/day for periods of 2-3 months. The therapy was supplemented by topical use of the drug in affected areas along with exposure to U.V. light. It is interesting to note that in one study,[15] opposite effects of topical and oral use of the drug were reported. According to this report, oral use decreased the erythema response of patients to ultraviolet light whereas the local application increased this response. The active principles were used at much lower doses, i.e. 5-20 mg/kg/day. The success of therapy in most of the reports was 70-80%. Some workers[16] reported that young patients responded more rapidly to therapy than the older patients, while others[18] found equal effect in all patients, irrespective of age, sex or duration of illness.

Mechanism of Action

The precise mechanism of action of *Ammi majus* in leucoderma is yet to be elucidated. Whether the furocoumarins elicit a direct action on Tyrosinase enzyme or affect the same indirectly is disputed. Lerner et al[15] reported that some irradiation products of psoralen interact with SH-groups which are inhibitory to Tyrosinase, U.V. light or solar irradiation act only as potentiators of psoralen effect.[19-21] 8-methoxypsoralen (Ammoidin) together with photo-oxidation of inhibitors and change in redox potential makes the conditions more favourable for normal melanin formation. The drug thus acts principally by photosensitizing action of its furocoumarins or their flourescent products.[22-24]

Epicutaneous application of furo-coumarins provokes dermatitis characterised by a latent period of erythema and later pigmentation. The part exposed to sunlight or U.V. light absorbs more rays after application of the drug facilitating normal pigmentation[25]. Chakraborty et al[26] and Biswas et al[27,28] demonstrated increased pigmentation in hypo-physectomised toads kept in darkness. Their results thus establish direct action of the drug on Tyriosinase without the involvement of melanophore stimulating hormone and U.V. light. Recent studies of Biswas *et al*[29] confirm the activation of Tyrosinase or its precursors by psoralen.

The present state of knowledge regarding the mechanism of action of *Ammi majus* was reviewed by Zafarullah and Vohora[2].

i. The action is through furocoumarins.

ii. Tyrosinase activity is affected by the drug. Whether this action is direct or indirect through participation of other factors, e.g., MSH, U.V. light, etc., is disputed. There is more evidence for a direct action.

iii. Role of solar/U.V. irradiation potentiates the action of the drug. The involvement of these factors is not essential.

Toxicity

A single dose of 400 mg/kg of xanthotoxin or imperatonin has been reported to be lethal in guinea pigs with lesions in liver and kidneys[30]. Chronic administration of the drug (1-2 mg/kg/day for 5 months) resulted in liver necrosis in young guinea pigs without affecting growth[31].

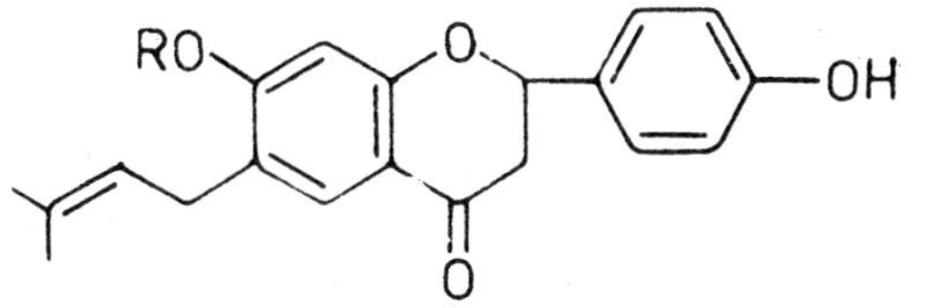

Bavachinin
R = Me
Bavachin
R = H

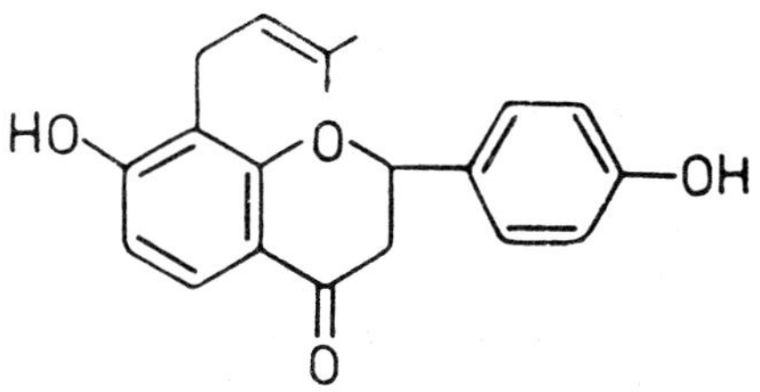

Isobavachin

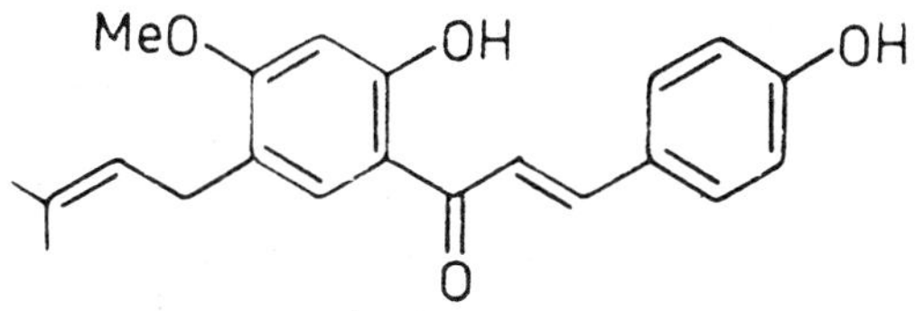

Bavachalcone

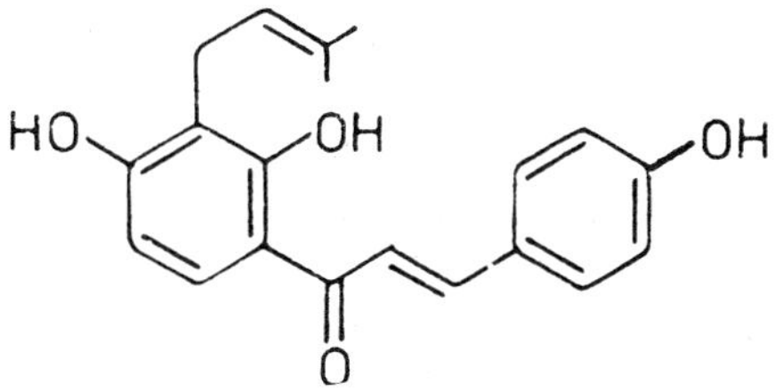

Isobavachalcone

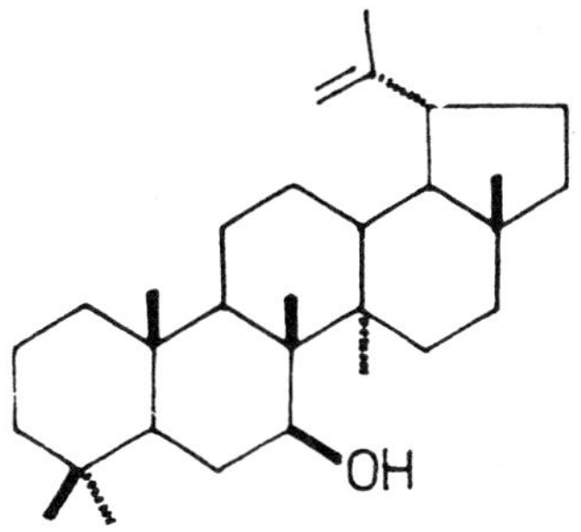

Psoracinol

Fig. 6.3 Some chemical principles isolated from *Psoralea corylifolia*.

6.4.2 *Psoralea corylifolia* Linn.

Chemistry

The plant is called *Babchi* in Ayurveda and its seeds are reputed for the treatment of leucoderma and bilious affections. Its traditional use in this disease stimulated researchers to undertake extensive chemical investigations. These have been reviewed thoroughly[12,13,32] and so have not been included here. Medicinally important chemical principles include psoralen, isopsoralen, corylifolean, angelicin bakuchiol, bavachin, bavachinin, isobavachin, bavachalcone, isobavachalcone, bavachromene, corylin, corylidin, corylinal, neobavaiso-flavone, psorolenol etc. Some of these are shown in Fig. 6.3.

Pharmacology and Mechanism of Action

Aqueous and ethanolic extracts and volatile oil have been reported to possess antibacterial, antifungal, antiviral, antiprotozoal, and anthelmintic actions both *in vitro* and *in vivo*. Isoproralen and angelicin revealed tranquillosedative, anticonvulsant and muscle relaxant properties in experimental animals while bavachinine showed anti-inflammatory effects. These have been reviewed by Satyavati and Coworkers[32].

Its principal action viz on pigment production has been extensively investigated at the Central Drug Research Institute, Lucknow. Furanocoumarins are known to be inactive *per se* but are activated following exposure to ultra violet light. Irradiation of psoralen with UV light (in the presence or absence of cysteine or other SH-compounds) leads to the formation of new fluorescent compounds quite different from the parent compound. Rashid Ali and Agarwala[33] showed that solar irradiation of psoralen in aqueous ethanol solution resulted in the formation of degradation products which have the capacity to inactivate SH-group. This was evident from its inhibitory effect on succinic dehydrogenase enzyme of rat kidney and reversal of thiourea inhibition by potato tyrosinase. It was postulated that pigment formation by psoralen may depend on the interaction of irradiated psoralen with SH groups which are inhibitory to tyrosinase. These workers also showed that psoralen significantly accelerates the photooxidation of dihydroxyphenylalanine (DOPA) under sun light, white light, and short wave UV light irradiation. It was found that SH compounds could inhibit psoralen-catalysed photooxidation of DOPA. The process was fasciliated by ascorbic acid and high pH. Possibly through accumulation in melanocytes, psoralen photooxidised the available DOPA to melanin, resulting in increased melanin formation[34].

Chakraborty and coworkers[35] reported that psoralen reduced hepatic ascorbic acid levels and accelerated skin melanogenesis in toads. They also described a useful method for the bioassay of psoralen and other drug used in leucoderma[36].

Clinical Studies

Many clinical reports are available on the efficacy of *P. corylifolia* powdered seeds, extracts, oil and active principles (particularly psoralen and isopsoralen) in leucoderma[5,9,10,37-40]. The drugs have been used both orally and by topical application. In studies carried out at CDRI, Lucknow and Christian Medical College, Vellore mixture of psoralen-isopsoralen, administered at 10-30 mg/kg/day alongwith local application gave very good results within 1-4 months. The recovery of pigment could be enhanced by 2-3 min exposure to UV light from mercury vapour lamps[37]. Better results were claimed by psoralen-trioxɛ ᴇn mixture[40]. In a recent study[10] fifty patients were treated with

8-methoxypsoralen at the All India Institute of Medical Sciences, New Delhi with very encouraging results. The drug was administered at 600 µg/kg p.o on alternate days followed by 2 h exposure to UV light ($0.5\text{-}5$ J/cm^2) for 9 months or till complete clearance occurred. The patients showed 25-83% repigmentation over a period of 77 treatment sessions.

Toxicity

The drugs psoralen/isopsoralen are fairly safe as indicated by little toxicity in studies on rats and guinea pigs. Isopsoralen exhibited no hepatotoxic effects in liver function tests in rabbits. Hepatotoxic action was, however, observed with imperatonin. The drugs revealed no evidence of teratogenic effects in experimental animals. Oral administration of seed powder elicits some undesirable side effects e.g. nausea, vomiting, and headache. Some local irritation may be observed on chronic topical use[32].

6.4.3 Other Plants and Formulations

Encouraging clinical results were reported with the use of medicinal plants *Semecarpus anacardium*[9]. *Ficus hispida*[41] and *Ficus tsiela*[42], Ayurvedic patent and coded drugs *Shashikala Vati*, CRIA-9, Ayush-57, *P. corylifolia* + *Gandhak Rasayana*, Unani coded drugs BS$_1$ to BS$_{10}$ and their combinations[43-45].

6.5 ROLE OF ELEMENTS

At least six elements (Al, Au, Cu, Fe, Hg and S) may be linked to this disease as follows:

6.5.1 Aluminum (Al)

In Unani medicine *Geru* (red ochre which contains Al silicate) is used (both orally and locally) for the treatment of leucoderma.[7]

6.5.2 Copper (Cu)

Copper has a special role in vitiligo or leucoderma. Though the precise etiology is not fully understood, the disease is attributed to disturbance in the synthesis of melanin and involves tyrosinase-a Cu containing enzyme[2]. Tahera and Qamaruddin[46] studied serum Cu levels in 55 normal subjects and 525 vitiligo patients. Their results, given below, indicate considerable elevation in serum Cu levels in this disease:

Group	Serum Cu (µg %) Mean ± S.D.	
	Male	**Female**
Normal subjects	69.3 ± 7.3	123.3 ± 26.8
Vitiligo patients	167.8 ± 45.0	152.7 ± 52.0

Paradoxically inorganic Cu salts (e.g. chloride and sulphate) and Cu containing plants (please see S. No. 21, 64, 68, 113, 128, 160, 181, 207, 227, 231 in Table 6.1) have also been used for the treatment of leucoderma in Unani[7] and Siddha[8] systems of medicine. Behl[5] reported lower serum Cu values in vitiligo patients and advocated the use of Cu chloride orally 1-3 mg/day in capsules or 200 µg i.v. twice a week for the treatment of this disease. Rashid Ali and Agarwal[47] studied the effect of feeding psoralen (a plant principle used in Vitiligo) on the Cu content of different organs in albino rats. Sivaprakasham and associates[48] conducted a clinical study in patients of leucoderma with a Siddha medicine called *Pennimelai Chendooram*. It is prepared from Cu pyrites rich in Fe. The authors reported complete relief in 5.7%, marked relief in 8.5%, and moderate relief in 11.42% cases. They remarked that while there are several theories and concepts regarding the etiology and pathogenesis of leucoderma, the medicine was probably effective in those cases where there was decrease in blood Cu, Fe and other trace elements.

6.5.3 Gold (Au)

In Siddha medicine Au preparations (*Swarn Bhasma, Agasthi–Aparipoornam 400 and Vaithia Poornam 250*) containing herbaturated Au oxide are described as remedies for leucoderma[8].

6.5.4 Iron (Fe)

Studies on 500 cases of vitiligo and 50 control subjects revealed significantly elevated serum Fe levels in the former[49]. Paradoxically the use of *Geru* (which contains FeO) has been described in the treatment of this disease.[7]

6.5.5 Mercury (Hg)

Mercury vapour lamps are used to produce VU light indicated in the treatment of leucoderma[5].

6.5.6 Sulphur (S)

It is advocated for the treatment of leucoderma in the form of copper sulphate[7] and *Gandhak Rasayana*[32].

6.6 ANIMAL ORIGIN DRUGS

Vohora and Khan[50] documented 20 drugs of animal origin with claimed efficacy in leucoderma (Table 6.2). These claims have not been validated by scientific investigations.

Table 6.2 Animal origin drugs mentioned in Unani texts as curative for leucoderma[50].

S.No.	Scientific Name (English Name)	Unani Name	Remarks
1.	*Python reticulatus* (Python)	Azdah	Live python is burnt and ash is mixed with honey for external application on patches.
2.	*Capra hircus* (Goat)	Bakra	Kidneys are given orally.
3.	*Pholeus herbraeves* *Vespa orientalis* (Yellow Wasp)	Bhid or Tataiya	Live wasps are made to sting the affected part. The wasps ground with honey and salt form a useful application for the treatment of this disease.

(Contd.)

4.	Class : *Archnida* N.O. : *Scorpiones* Many species (Scorpion)	Bichhoo	Dried scorpions are pulverized and mixed with vinegar for application on leucoderma/vitiligo and alopecia.
5.	*Milvus migrans* (Pariah Kite)	Cheel	Eggs are boiled in oil to form a useful application for leucoderma patches.
6.	*Talpa micrura* (Mole or Shrew)	Chhahoondar	Flesh with rose oil is used for external application.
7.	*Bos taurus* (Cow)	Gai	Brain is minced and mixed with vinegar for external application.
8.	*Calumba livia* (Blue Rock Pigeon)	Kabootar	Excreta is used for topical application
9.	*Cyprea moneta* (Crowrie)	Kauri	Local application of powder or ash of yellow variety with salt petre.
10.	*Scilla serrata* (Crab)	Kekra or Sartan	Ash is applied on patches.
11.	*Oryctolagus cuniculus* (Rabbit)	Khargosh	Fresh blood forms a useful application.
12.	*Grus grus lilfordi* (Eastern crane)	Kulang	Brain is made into a paste and applied on affected parts.
13.	*Pisces* (Fish)	Machhli	Ash of bones forms a useful external application.
14.	*Crocodilus polustris* (Crocodile)	Magarmachh	Blood with other medicaments is applied on vitiligo patches.
15.	*Musca domestica* (House Fly)	Makkhi	Excreta is used externally.
16.	*Pavo cristatus* (Peacock)	Mor	Ash of bones is applied on affected parts.
17.	*Melursus ursinus* (Bear)	Reechh	Fat is applied on patches.
18.	Class : *Reptilia* N.O. : *Ophidia* many species (snake)	Saanp	Whole eviscerated snake is stuffed with leaves of *Fumaria offcinalis* and sutured. It is then put in hot ash. Well cooked leaves are removed, pulverized and applied on affected parts. This treatment is claimed to cure leucoderma within 24 h. Local application of snake castings, ash of black snake and snake eggs with vinegar.
19.	From the stomach of *Acipenser huso* (Isinglass)	Saresham Mahi	Isinglass (a finely shredded and dried secretion from the stomach of some fishes) is claimed to be of value is leucoderma.
20.	An aquatic bird found near river banks. It produces *Waque, Waque* sound; hence the name	Waque	Bile is applied externally.

6.7 REFERENCES

1. Dutta AK and Mandal SB (1980) *Proceedings of the Seminar on Bars (Leucoderma)*, pp. 16-23, New Delhi; Central Council for Research in Unani Medicine.

2. Zafarullah M and Vohora SB (1980) *Ibid.*, pp. 125-131.

3. Meister A (1950) *Biochemistry of Amino Acids*, ed. 2, Vol. 2, p. 920, New York: Academic Press.

4. Mukherjee GD (1980) *Proceedings of the Seminar on Bars (Leucoderma)*, pp. 97-100, New Delhi: Central Council for Research in Unani Medicine.

5. Behl PN, Arora RB, and Srivastava G (1992) *Traditional Indian Dermatology: Concepts Past and Present*, pp. 15, 17, 47, 48, 69, 70, 96, 111, New Delhi: Skin Institute and School of Dermatology.

6. Mitra R and Pandey HC (1980) *Proceedings of the Seminar on Bars (Leucoderma)*, pp. 132-141, New Delhi: Central Council for Research in Unani Medicine.

7. Khan MMA, Zohra A and Bano M (1980), *Ibid*, pp. 169-176.

8. Kumaraswamy R. Joseph MA, Nathan EM et al (1980) *Ibid*, pp. 169-176.

9. Anonymous (1984) *Ayurvedic Research Seminar on Skin Diseases*, Abstract Book, pp. 7-11, Jamnagar: Gujarat Ayurved University.

10. Kumar S, Kumar VS, Sharma A et al eds. (1994) *Traditional Medicinal Plants in Skin Care*, Lucknow: Central Institute of Medicinal and Aromatic Plants.

11. Fowlks WN (1959) *J Invest Dermatol* **32**, 249.

12. Rastogi RP and Mehrotra BN (1991) *Compendium of Indian Medicinal Plants*, vol. 1, pp. 9-31, 332-333, Lucknow: Central Drug Research Institute and New Delhi: Publication and Information Directorate.

13. Rastogi RP and Mehrotra BN (1991) *Compendium of Indian medicinal Plants* Vol. 2, pp. 38-39, 567, 568, Lucknow: Central Drug Research Institute and New Delhi: Publication and Information Directorate.

14. El Mofty AM (1952) *Brit J Dermatol* **64**, 431.

15. Lerner AB, Denton CR and Fitzpatrik TB (1953) *J Invest Dermatol* **20**, 299.

16. Fitztrik TB, Arsdt KA, El-Mofty AM et al (1966) *Arch Dermatol* **20**, 299.

17. Saleem Y, Hussain SMS, Siddiqui MA et al (1976) *J Res Indian Med Yoga Homeo* **11(2)**, 75.

18. Hussain SMS, Kazmi SHT and Taiyab HM (1978) *J Res Indian Med Yoga Homeo* **13(1)**, 1.

19. Shareef MA, Lateef A, Hussain A et al (1987) *First Internat Seminar Unani Medicine,* New Delhi: Council for Research in Unani Medicine.

21. Fitzpatrick, TB, Hopkins, CB, Bleikenstaff, DD et al. (1955) *J. Invest. Derm.*, **25**, 187.

22. Arnold, HN (1957) *Hawai Med. J.* **10**, 391.

23. Becker, SW (1958) *Science*, **12**, 878.

24. Pathak, MA, Feliman, JH and Kanfuran, KD (1960) *J. Invest, Derm.*, **35**, 165.

25. Musajo, L, Rodighiero G and Dall Acqua, I (1965) *Experimental*, **21**, 24.

26. Musajo, L and Rodigheiron G (1962), *Experimental*, **18**, 153.

27. Kelly, FE and Pinkus, H (1955) *J. Invest Derm.*, **25**, 453.

28. Chakraborty, DP, Deb, C and Mukerjee, M (1959), *Sci. Cult*, **25**, 386.

29. Biswas, NM Chakraborty, DP and Deb, C *Naturwissench*, **22**, 622.

30. Biswas, NM, Deb, C Haque, M and Chakraborty, DP (1967) *Endocrinoligie*, **52**, 271.

31. Chakraborty, DP Roychoudhary SK and Dey RN (1976), *Clinika Chemica Acta*, **72**, 219.

32. Satyavati GV, Gupta AK and Tandon N (1987) *Medicinal Plants of India*, vol. 2,pp. 518-530, New Delhi: Indian Council of Medical Research.

33. Rashid Ali and Agarwala SC (1962), *J Sci Industr Res*, **21C**, 321.

34. Rashid Ali and Agarwala SC (1965) *Indian J Biochem*, **2**, 271.

35. Chakraborty DP, Roychowdhury SK and Dey RN (1978), *Sci Cult*, **44**, 321.

36. Chakraborty DP, Chatterjee A., Chakraborty AK et al (1981) *Sci Cult* **47**, 228.

37. Mukherji B (1956) *J Sci Industr Res*, **15A(5) Suppl.**, 1.

38. Chakravarti RN, Chakravorty AN, Rao A et al (1956) *Bull Calcutta Sch Trop Med* **4**, 175.

39. Singh, RN and Chaturvedi GN (1966) *Indian J Dermatol Venerol*, **32**, 113.

40. Sehgal VN, Rege VL, and Kharangate VN (1978), *Int J Dermatol*, **17**, 243.

41. Trivedi VP, Ansari Z and Shukla K (1980), *Proceedings Seminar on Bars (Leucoderma)*, pp. 68-77, New Delhi: Central Council for Research in Unani medicine.

42. Jopat PD and Karnick CR (1980) *Ibid*, pp. 83-86.

43. Ahmad M, Waheed MA, Khan MMA et al (1987) *First International Seminar on Unani Medicine*, Abstract Book, p. 26, New Delhi: Central Council for Research in Unani Medicine and WHO.

44. Ansari KB, Ahmad A., Noor A et al (1987) *Ibid* p. 26.

45. Khan MA, Khan SSA, Husain SMS et al (1987) *Ibid*, p. 27.

46. Tahera SS and Qamaruddin S (1980) *Proceedings Seminar on Bars* (Leucoderma), pp. 165-168, New Delhi: Central Council for Research in Unani Medicine.

47. Rashid Ali and Agarwala SC (1969) *Experientia* **25**, 24.

48. Sivaprakasam K, Anandan T, Yashodha R et al (1987) *Second World Congress on Yoga and Ayurveda*, Abstract Book, p. 120, Varanasi: Banaras Hindu University.

49. Tahera SS (1980) *Second Scientific Seminar of CCRUM*, Abstract Book p. 12, New Delhi: Central Council for Research in Unani Medicine.

50. Vohora SB and Khan MSY (1978) *Animal Origin Drugs used in Unani Medicine* pp. 87, 88, New Delhi: Institute of History of Medicine and Medical Research and Vikas Publishing House Pvt. Ltd.

7

Leprosy

7.1 LEPROSY: AYURVEDIC AND UNANI CONCEPTS

Leprosy is a dreadful crippling disease afflicting about 15 million people in the world, of which about one third are in India[1], with widespread ulcerous lesions which in severe cases may result in sloughing of fingers, toes and limbs. The disease is fatal when it affects vital organs. High morbidity, chronic course, social stigma and humiliation cause serious psychological damage in the victims, thus making their lives miserable. The disease, as we know it today, is caused by *Mycobacterium leprae*. Though modern drugs e.g. dapsone, rifampin and clofazimine have made a definite place in the treatment of leprosy and accompanying tuberculous complications, we do not have an ideal drug for treating this disease. A study of traditional concepts may be helpful in better understanding and therapy of leprosy.

Kusht Rog (Leprosy) has been described in ancient Ayurvedic texts since Vedic age (5000 BC) and was known to be a major health problem at the time of Charaka and Sushruta (300-500 BC). These ancient physicians clearly mentioned that the disease was due to the presence of *doshas* (impurities) and *krimi* (bacteria) and other etiological factors. They used a wide range of herbs, minerals, *Shodhna* (elimination) and *panchkarma* (five procedure) therapy for the management of leprosy[2,3]. In Unani (Greco-Arabian) medicine *Juzam* (leprosy) is believed to be caused by infiltration and dispersal of *sauda* (burnt humours) throughout the body disturbing the normal temperament of the organs. *Sauda* is produced by the burning of *balgam* (phelgm), safra (bile) and *khoon* (blood). Excessive *sauda* production or retention in the body may be due to the following causes[4].

i. Disturbance in the temperament of the liver causing increase in heat and dryness resulting in excessive burning of humours.

ii. Excessive coldness in the temperament and consequent concentration of blood.

iii. Food producing more *sauda* (burnt humours) and *balgam* (phelgm), e.g. fish or foul meat.

iv. Obstruction of passage of blood towards the spleen preventing the separation of *sauda* (burnt humour) from *khoon* (blood).

v. Weak expelling power of the rectum, kidneys, uterus and skin, causing accumulation of burnt humours.

vi. Obstruction of skin pores preventing heat loss.

vii. Causes enumerated in v and vi above make the subject more prone to infections from other patients and the atmosphere.

viii. Hereditary factors.

Unani-Tibb also utilizes natural products: drugs of plant, mineral and animal origin for the treatment of leprosy.

7.2 PLANT, MINERAL AND ANIMAL ORIGIN DRUGS

Zafarullah and coworkers[5] and Vohora and Khan[6] presented lists of plant, mineral and animal origin drugs used in the treatment of leprosy alongwith their doses and methods of administration (Tables 7.1-7.3). Single drugs are seldom used in these systems. Polypharmacy employing formulations containing a large number of simples is mainly practiced. Some of the compound prescriptions commonly used in Unani-Tibb for the treatment of this disease are shown in Table 7.4.

Table 7.1 Plant Drugs used for the Treatment of Leprosy[5]

Botanical Name (Unani Name)	Part (s) Used	Mode of Administration	Doses/Day
Aconitum ferox (Bish)	Roots	Oral	2-4 g
Albizzia lebbeck (Siras)	Stem bark	Oral and as an external application of the decoction	5-7 g
Azadirachta indica (Neem)	Leaves & fruits	Dried plant material is mixed with mustard oil and applied on lesions	—
Calortropis procera (Madar)	Root bark	Oral	0.5 g
Convolvulus arvensis (Hirankhuri)	Whole plant	Orally with black pepper	5-10 g
Eclipta alba (Bhanghrah)	Leaves	Oral	5-10 g
Gynocardia odorata (Chaulmogra)	Seeds	Oil used both orally and as an external application	5-10 drops. Up to 30 drops in severe cases
Smilax chinensis (Chob chini)	Roots	Decoction orally	5-10 g
Sphaeranthus indicus (Mundi)	Flowers	Oral	10 g
Swertia chirata (Chiraita)	Whole plant	Decoction, oral	5-7 g
Trichosanthes cordata (Pathal)	Roots	Oral	3 g

N.B. : Dried pulverized plant material is used as such except where it is mentioned otherwise.

Table 7.2 Mineral Drugs used for the treatment of Leprosy[5]

English Name/Composition	Unani Name	Mode of Administration	Dose/Day
Arsenic	Sankhia	Oral use as well as local application. Kushta, Safuf & Johar for oral use. Ointments for local application.	1-5 mg
Lapis laziole	Lajward	Orally in compound preparations	1-2 mg
Arsenic trisulphide	Hartal	Oral use in the form of Kushta & Safuf	20-25 mg
Silicate of aluminia & iron oxide	Geru	Oral and local use	1-3 g
Sulphur	Gandhak	Oral and local use in compound preparations	500-700 mg
Cinnabar	Shangraf	Orally	10-15 mg

Table 7.3 Animal origin drugs used for the treatment of Leprosy[5,6]

Scientific Name	Unani Name (English Name)	Part Used	Mode of Administration
a) *Daboia russel Vel elegans* b) *Echis carinata*	Aphai (Viper)	Flesh cooked with olive oil, salt and *Anethum sowa*	Orally
Not available	Azfrul teep (a sea shell)	Powder	Orally
Bos bubalus	Bhains (Buffalo)	Freshly butchered eviscerated animal	Sitting inside the abdominal cavity
Ovis vignei	Bhed (Sheep)	Urine	External application
Leptoptilos dubius	Dheenk (Adjutant stork)	Eggs	Orally
Elephus maximus	Haathi (Elephant)	Fine powder or ash of ivory	Both orally and as an external application
Calumba livia	Kabootar (Pigeon)	Flesh	Orally
From insect *Coccus lacca*	Lakh (Lac)	Powder	External application
Corallium rubrum	Marjan (Coral)	Powder	External application
Pincatada	Moti (Pearls)	Ash	Orally
Camelus dromedarius	Oont (Camel)	Curd	Orally
Class : *Reptilia* N.O. : *Ophidia* Many species	Saanp (Snake)	a) Slough with grams b) Venom	Orally

(Contd.)

Hystrix indica	Sehi (Indian porcupine)	Flesh	Orally
Mel	Shehd (Honey)	—	Orally
Panthera tigris	Sher (Tiger)	Fat	External application
a) *Locusta migratoria* b) *Schistocerca gregaria*	Tiddi (Locust)	Whole organism	Orally

Table 7.4 Compound Formulations used in Unani medicine for the Treatment of Leprosy[5]

Receipe	Method of Preparation	Mode of Administration	Dose/Day
1. HAB-I-JUZAM: Poast-i-Bikh-i-Madar (*Calotropis gigantea*, root bark) : 4 kg Wheat : 250 g Water : q.s.	Plant material is soaked over-night in water. Next day wheat encapsulated in cloth pouch is soaked in this infusion. The whole container is then dumped under elephant or horse dung. After 28 days the container is taken out, water evaporated. Wheat pounded into fine powder and 61 pills are made from the powder.	Orally with wheat bread and Ghee (clarified butter)	1 pill
2. KUSHTA-I-HARTAL: a) Hartal Warqi (Arsenic sulphide) : 10 g b) Magz-Karanjwa (*Caesalpinia bonducella* seed kernel) : 20 g c) Nagphani/Sphutica (*Opuntia vulgaris*, stem) : 20 g	Ingredients a & b pulverized. Drugs arranged in earthen vessel in layers in following order from below upward: 1. Karanjwa, 2. Nagphani, 3. Hartal, 4. Nagphani, 5. Karanjwa. Vessel then covered with mud plaster, dried & placed in cow dung fuel pit to make the Kushta by Gil-Hikmat process. Powder is stored in airtight bottles.	Orally	Equivalent to 4 rice grains (64 rice grains = 1g)
3. MAJUN-I-JUZAM: Badyan (*Foenculum vulgare*) : 25 g Bisfaiz (*Polypodium vulgare*) : 25 g Bahera (*Terminalla belerica*) : 25 g Poast Drakht Anjir (*Ficus carica*) : 50 g	All ingredients are pulverized and sieved through 80 mesh sieve. White sugar made into Qiwam (hot thick syrup) and the above powder gradually added to it stirring constantly. Majun so prepared is stored in glass jars.	Orally-before breakfast with water	10 g

(Contd.)

Poast Darakht Nim
(*Azadirachta indica*
bark)   : 100 g

Poast Halilah-i-Zard
(*Terminalla chebula,*
fruit peel)   : 25 g

Shahtrah (*Fumaria
officinalis*)   : 25 g

Kishiz Kushk (*Coriandrum
sativum*)   : 25 g

Chiraita Talkh
(*Swertia chirata*)   : 25 g

Chita Lakri (*Plumbago
zeylanica*)   : 25 g

Darunaj Aqrabi
(*Doronicum hookeri*) : 25 g

Sana-i-Makki (*Cassia
angustifolia*)   : 25 g

Gul-i-Surkh
(*Rosa damascena*)   : 25 g

Halilal-i-Siah
(*Terminalia chebula*) : 25 g

Qiwam Shakar Safaid
(White sugar syrup)   : 1.5 kg

4. MAJUN USHBAH: As in Recipe 3   As in Recipe 3   5-10 g
   Amla (*Emblica
   officinalis*)   : 25 g

Aftimoon (*Cuscuta
spp.*)   : 300 g

Burada Sandal Surkh
(*Pterocarpus
santalinus*)   : 50 g

Badyan (*Foeniculum
vulgare*)   : 100 g

Balchhar (*Valeriana
officinalis*)   : 50 g

(*Contd.*)

Bisfaij (*Polypodium vulgare*) : 100 g

Bahera (*Terminalia belerica*) : 20 g

Poast-Halilah-i-Zard (*Terminalia chebula*, Peel) : 25 g

Chob Chini (*Smilax china*) : 150 g

Darchini (*Cinnamomum officinalis*) : 50 g

Sann-i-Makki (*Cassia angustifolia*) : 200 g

Shahtrah (*Fumaria officinalis*) : 50 g

Ushbah Maghrabi (*Smilax officinalis*) : 200 g

Kabab Chini (*Piper cubeba*) : 50 g

Gul-i-Surkh (*Rosa damascena*) : 100 g

Qiwam Shakar Safaid (White sugar syrup) : 4.6 kg

5. SAFUF HARTAL: Hartal Warqi (Arsenic trisulphide) : 10 g Filfil Siah (*Piper nigrum*) : 21 fruits	Two ingredients are powdered together	Orally in Pan (*Piper betle*, leaf)	1-2 Ratti (8 Ratti = 1 g)	
6. SAFUF MUBARAK: Poast-i-Halilah-i-Zard (*Terminalia chebula*, fruit peel) : 2 g	Powdered and seived	Orally	0.5 g	

Poast Bahera (*Terminalia belerica*, fruits) : 2 g

Amla (*Emblica officinalis*, fruits) : 2 g

Gul-i-Surkh (*Rosa damascena*, flowers) : 1 g

(*Contd.*)

Sat-i-Giloe (*Tinospora cordifolia* extract)   : 1 g

Revand Chini (*Rheum emodi*, rhizomes)   : 1 g

Mulethi (*Glycyrrhiza glabra*, root)   : 1 g

Chob Chini (*Smilax chinensis*, root)   : 1 g

Chhoti Eleichi (*Cardamomum officinalis* fruits)   : 1 g

Dhania Khushk (*Coriandrum sarivum*, fruits)   : 1 g

Geru (a kind of clay)   : 1 g

Poast Tewaj Khatai (*Wrightia antidysentrica*, stem bark)   : 1 g

Anjir Jungli ki Jar (*Ficus spicata*, root bark)   : 1 g

Poast Bikh Anjir Jungli (*Ficus spicata*, root bark)   : 1 g

Panwad (*Cleome brachycarpa*, seeds)   : 1 g

Sarphooka (*Tephrosea purpurea* whole plant)   : 1 g

Tukhm-i-Babchi (*Psoralea corylifolia*, seeds)   : 1 g

Neem (*Azadirachta indica,* leaves flowers, fruits)   : 1 g of each

Gandhak (Sulphur)   : 0.5 g

(*Contd.*)

7. SHARBAT-I-UNNAB MURAKKAB:

a) Unnab (*Ziziphus sativas*, fruits) : 20 fruits

b) Gul-i-Banafsha (*Viola odorata*, flowers) : 8 g

c) Gul-i-Nilofar (*Nymphaea alba*, flowers) : 8 g

d) Gul-i-Gaozban (*Caccinia glauca*, flowers) : 8 g

e) Gulab (*Rosa damascena*, flowers) : 8 g

f) Arq-i-Gulab (Aqua *Rosa domascena*) : 3 l

g) Arq-i-Bed Mushk (Aqua *Salix capraea*) : 3 l

h) Turanjbin (*Hedysarum alhagi*, gum) : 0.5 kg

i) Shirkhisht (*Fraxinus ornus*, latex) : 0.5 kg

j) Sugar : 0.5 kg

Ingredients a-g boiled and concentrated until the volume is reduced to 1.5 liters. Then ingredients h-j added and heated sufficiently to make the Qiwam.

Orally

5-10 g.

8. TIRYAQ-ARBAAH:
a) Habul Ghar (*Laurus nobilis*, fruits) : q.s.

b) Mur Maki (*Balsamodendron myrrh*, resin) : q.s.

c) Juntiana (*Bergenia ligulata*, roots) : q.s.

d) Zarawand (*Aristolochia indica*, rhizomes) : q.s.

e) Honey : q.s.

Ingredients a-d powdered, sieved and mixed with honey in sufficient quantity to make the Majun. Should be used after 40 days of preparation. The majun is effective up to two years after preparation.

Orally

4-5 g

(Contd.)

9. TIRYAQ-I-FAROOQ:

a) Ajmud (*Apium graveolens*) : 15 g

b) Ajwain Desi (*Prychotis ajowan*) : 15 g

c) Azkhar Makki (*Cymbopogon schoenanthus*) : 15 g

d) Ustukhuddus (*Lavandula stoechas*) : 15 g

e) Aqaqin (*Acacia arabica*) : 10 g

f) Anusun (*Pimpinella anisum* whole extract of plant) : 10 g

g) Badyan (*Foeniculum vulgare*) : 10 g

h) Irisa (*Iris florentina*) : 30 g

i) Gul-i-Bansal (*Amomum racemosum*, flowers) : 10 g

j) Loban (*Boswellia serrata*) : 15 g

k) Gorakmundi (*Sphaeranthus indicus*) : 30 g

l) Mushktara Mushi (*Mentha sylvestris*) : 15 g

m) Mastage (*Pistacia lentiscus*) : 15 g

n) Balchar, Nardin (*Valeriana officinalis*) : 15 g

o) Gond Kikar (*Acacia arabica* gum) : 10 g

p) Guggul (*Balsamodendron gugul*) : 5 g

q) Qurs-i-Afai (Tablets made from viper flesh and wheat flour) : 120 g

All dry constituents are mixed, triturated, sieved through mesh number 60 and made into a Sufuf. Garlic ground separately in orange juice and filtered through a cloth. The remaining Sharab and the ground garlic are mixed with the Sufuf. When it dries, ingredients q-s added to it after being pulverized to fine grains. Powder is again sieved through sieve number 60. During the preparation of the Qiwam of honey, it is essential to add "u". After the Qiwam has been removed from the fire, saffron ground in "x" is added to it. To the semi-hot Qiwam the Sufuf is gradually added with agitation. The preparation of the Tiryaq is complete when a compatible mixture forms.

Orally, should 1 g be used with Dawaul-Misk and Khamira Gaozaban Ambari.

(*Contd.*)

r) Sharab-i-Santra (Orange
juice)   : 750 ml

s) Lahsan (*Allium sativum*) : 60 g

t) Roghan-i-Balsam (Oil of
*Balsamodendron
opobalsamus*)   : 30 g

u) Zafran (*Crocus sativus*) : 30 g

v) Ghee (Clarified butter)   : 4 g

w) Arq-i-Gaozahan (Aqua
Onosma bracteatum)   : 50 ml

10. TIRYAQ ZAHAB

   Moti (Pearl)   : q.s.

   Ailwa (*Aloe vera*,
   extract)   : 35 g

   Siqmonia (*Convovulus
   scamonia*, resin)   : 35 g

   Aftimoon (*Cuscuta* spp.,
   whole plant)   : 18 g

   Darchini (*Cassia
   cinnamon*, bark)   : 18 g

   Chiraita (*Swertia chirata*
   whole plant)   : 18 g

   Laung (*Caryophylus
   aromaticus*, flower buds) : 15 g

   Ud-Hindi (*Aquilaria
   agallocha*, wood)   : 15 g

   Lajward (Lapis lazuli,
   stone)   : 15 g

   Sandal Surkh (*Pterocarpus
   santalinus*, wood)   : 15 g

   Gond Katira (*Cochlospermum
   religiosum*, gum)   : 15 g

Pearls soaked in water in which Orally   5 g.
rice has been washed earlier. The
glass vessel containing the above
is then sealed with wax and
immersed in hot water for 3
weeks. Other ingredients are
pulverized and mixed in this
solution to yield a pasty material
from which pills are made. The
recommended size of the pills is
that of gram (*Cicer arietinum*)

(*Còntd.*)

11. ROGHAN AURAM SAUDVI:		The til oil is heated in an iron vessel. Other ingredients are	Applied locally
Phitkari (Alum)	: 10 g	pulverized separately. Alum is mixed gradually in the oil and	
Nila Tutiya (Copper sulphate)	: 10 g	stirred continuously with the help of a branch of Neem (*Azadirachra indica*) tree. Then the remining	
Sankhiya (Arsenic)	: 15 g	alum and arsenic are poured and mixed. The solution in oil is taken	
Til Oil (*Sesamum indicum*, oil)	: 120 g	from fire and stirred for 2 minutes more and preserved.	
12. ROGHAN JUZAM		Tablets made from ingredients (a) and (c) are boiled and burnt in Til	Applied on leprous ulcers.
a) Berge Mehndi (*Lawsonia inermis*, leaves)	: 500 g	oil successively with constant stirring. The oil is then filtered and is ready for use.	
b) Til Oil (*Seasamum indicum*, oil)	: 2 l		
c) Berge Neem (*Azadirachta indica*, leaves)	: 500 g		
13. ROGHAN QUST:		Ingredients a-c are boiled and burnt in oil (f) to form a poultice.	Luke-warm poultice is applied to affected parts.
a) Aqarqarha (*Anacyclus pyrethrum*, root)	: 8 g		
b) Filfil-i-Siah (*Piper nigrum*, fruit)	: 6 g		
c) Qust Talkh (*Saussurea lappa*)	: 180 g		
d) Farfi., (*Antiquorum exuda*)	: 6 g		
e) Jundb (*Castoreum*)	: 5 g		
f) Roghan Kunjad (*Sesamum indicum*, oil):	: 560 g		

7.3 SCIENTIFIC INVESTIGATIONS

A survey of of scientific work carried out in India[1,7-9] revealed that most of these drugs have not been investigated by experimental or clinical studies to confirm or refute their claimed efficacy in leprosy. A few clinical studies on some Ayurvedic plants, reputed to be useful in this disease, are however available. These include reports on *Achyranthes aspera*[10], *Alectra parasitica* (a parasitic plant found on the roots of *Vitex negundo*)[11-13], *Semecarpus anacardium*[14], *Acacia catechu*[3] and a compound drug *Arogyawardhini*[3]. Some of these reports do not conform to acceptable norms and international standards for clinical trials. This aspect warrants attention of competent and dedicated researchers to unearth useful antileprotic drugs from natural sources.

7.4 ELEMENTOLOGICAL APPROACH

Another aspect on which some pioneering work has been carried out at Jamia Hamdard is the elementological approach. The science of Medical Elementology believes that the key to all human ailments lies within us and involves restoration of a balanced state of elements. Infection upsets the homeostasis by the disease process *per se* or by the therapy adopted[15,16]. Vohora[17] carried out a survey of literature and reported that at least 16 elements (Al, As, Br, Ca, Co, Cr, Cu, Fe, Mg, N, Na, O, P, S, Sr and Zn) affect leprosy by virtue of changes in tissue/body fluid levels, therapeutic use and adverse effects.

Decreased levels of plasma/serum Ca, Fe, Mg, N, Na, P and Zn and increased serum Cu concentrations are observed in leprosy. This is probably true for all infectious diseases and has been attributed to increased urinary loss (Ca, Mg, N, Na, P, Zn) and a redistribution of these elements between blood and tissues. Skin Fe and Zn concentrations show a rise in leprosy. Clinical implications of these findings have not been explored.

At least seven elements (Al, As, Br, Fe, S, Sr and Zn) find therapeutic applications in leprosy. The preparations include Burrow's lotion, Fowler's solution, Ekzebrol (Strontium bromide), sulfones, inorganic S and Zn salts, adhesive Zn tape and variety of indigenous mineral preparations e.g. *Geru*(red ochre containing Fe oxide and Al silicate), *Jast* (Zn) and *Hartal / Sammul Far* (As sulphides) in the form of *Safuf* (fine powders) or *Kushtas / Bhasmas* (calcined metals) and ointments/lotions for external applications. An association between lepromatous leprosy and allergic contact dermatitis due to Cr in cement has been confirmed clinically and biologically in a male patient[18].

Details of the links of individual elements with this disease were reported earlier.[17] It is hoped that research on elementological aspects of leprosy may throw more light on the pathogenesis and therapy of this dreadful disease.

7.5 REFERENCES

1. *Central Drug Research Institute: R & D Highlights* (1991), p. 98, C.D.R.I., Lucknow.
2. Behl PN, Arora RB and Srivastava G (1992): *Traditional Indian Dermatology: Concepts of Past and Present*, pp. 38-47. New Delhi: Skin Institute and School of Dermatology.
3. *Ayurvedic Research Seminar on Skin Diseases* (1984): Gujarat Ayurved University, Jamnagar, Feb. 28 to March 1.
4. Avicenna SBA (1906): *Al Qanoon* (Arabic), Vol. 4, pp. 180-81, Lucknow: Matba-i-Nami.
5. Zafarullah M, Hassina Bano and Vohora SB (1980): *Amer J Chinese Med* **8(4)**, 370.
6. Vohora SB and Khan MSY (1978): *Animal Origin Drugs used in Unani Medicine*, pp. 86, 116-127, New Delhi: Institute of History of Medicine and Medical Research and Vikas Publishing House.
7. Satyavati GV, Raina MM and Sharma M (1976) *Medicinal Plants of India* Vol. 1, New Delhi: Indian Council of Medical Research.
8. Rastogi RP and Dhawan BN (1982) *Indian J Med Res* **76** (**Suppl.**), 27.
9. Satyavati GV, Gupta AK and Tandon N (1987). *Medicinal Plants of India* Vol. 2, New Delhi, Indian Council of Medical Research.
10. Ojha D. and Singh G (1968) *Lepr Rev.*, **39**, 23.
11. Prasad BN (1962) *Lepr Rev* **33**, 207.
12. Ghosh S and Chakravarty BK (1964). *Bull Calcutta Sch Trop Med* **12**, 179.
13. Bedi R (1968) *Ayurved Mahasammelan Patrika* **55**, 351.
14. Ojha D (1967) *Lepr India* **39**, 165.
15. Beisel WR (1972) *Amer J Clin Nutr* **25**, 1254.
16. Pandey VK, Parmeswaran M, Soman SD et al (1982) *Magnesium Bull* **2**, 141.
17. Vohora SB (1986) *Indian J Leprosy* **58(3)**, 451.
18. Jerez J, Quintanilla E, Martingil D et al (1980) *Dermatologica* **160**, 30.

8
Contributions from Jamia Hamdard

8.1 BOOKS/BOOK CHAPTERS

8.1.1 Waheed A and Siddiqui HH (1961) In *A Survey of Drugs*, pp. 118, 119, 140-148, 151-155, 163-166 New Delhi, Institute of History of medicine and Medical Research.

8.1.2 Vohora SB and Khan MSY (1978) In *Animal Origin Drugs used in Unani Medicine*, pp. 61-63, 74, 86, 87, 94, 101-103, 107-109, New Delhi, Institute of History of medicine and Medical Research and Vikas Publishing House.

8.1.3 Vohora SB (1980) Atrilal: A Unani drug for the treatment of *Bars Abyaz* (Vitiligo) with special reference to the possible mechanism of action. In: *Proceedings Seminar on Bars (Leucoderma)*, pp. 125-131, New Delhi, Central Council for Research in Unani Medicine.

8.1.4 Arora RB (1986) *Proceedings of the Symposium on Dermatology and Unani System of Medicine* (contributors from Jamia Hamdard: Abdul Hameed, Jameel Ahmad, SB Vohora, RB Arora, NI Ansari), H.N.F. Monograph No. 4, pp. 1-28, New Delhi, Hamdard National Foundation.

8.1.5 Vohora SB (1987) Elementology of leprosy. In: *Elements in Health and Disease*, (eds Said M, Rahman MA, D'Silva LA), pp. 586-593, Bait al-Hikmat Publication Series No. 1, Karachi Hamdard University Press.

8.1.6 Hamdard ME and Vohora SB (1989). Skin diseases, In: *Medical Elementology: Practical Applications*, pp. 8-10, New Delhi, Institute of History of Medicine and Medical Research.

8.1.7 Hameed A and Vohora SB (1990) Skin diseases. In: *New Horizons of Health Aspects of Elements*, Indo Polish Book (eds. Vohora SB and Dobrowolski JW) Chapter 5.3, pp. 163-176, New Delhi, Jamia Hamdard.

8.1.8 Athar M, Agarwal R, Bickers DR et al (1992) Pharmacological aspects of reactive oxygen species in skin In: *Pharmacology of Skin*, Florida, CRC Press.

8.1.9 Athar M and Vohora SB (1995). *Heavy Metals and Environment* pp. 30, 104-107, 166, 177, New Delhi. New Age International Ltd./Wiley Eastern Ltd.

8.1.10 Vohora SB and Vohora D (1997). *Skin care and herbomineral beauty aids in India. In: Women and Health : Ethnomedical Perspectives (Eds. Gottschalk-Batschkus CE, Schuler J and Iding D)*, pp. 125-132, Berlin, VWB.

8.2 Ph.D. THESES

8.2.1 Nanda A (1994) Development of transdermal drug delivery system by ionophoresis for some antihypertensive drugs and its evaluation. *Ph.D. Thesis*, New Delhi, Jamia Hamdard (Supervisor: RK Khar).

8.2.2 Giri U (1996) Role of free radicals in chemical carcinogenesis. *PhD. Thesis*, New Delhi, Jamia Hamdard (supervisor: M Athar)

8.2.3 Rezazadeh H (1996) Role of iron in the manefestation of chemical carcinagensis. *PhD. Thesis*, New Delhi (Supervisor : M Athar)

8.2.4 Khan HA (1996): Essential and toxic elements in food and feed arailable in Northern India: a model study of Delhi township. *PhD. Thesis*, New Delhi, Jamia Hamdard (Supervisor: M Athar).

8.3 M. PHARM THESES

8.3.1 Misra A (1989) Perforated film in the transdermal delivery of drugs. *M. Pharm Thesis*, New Delhi, Jamia Hamdard (Supervisor: RK Khar).

8.3.2 Asudani S (1991) Formulation and evaluation of polymer film laminates for transdermal use. *M. Pharm Thesis*, New Delhi, Jamia Hamdard (Supervisor: RK Khar).

8.3.3 Singh SJ (1992) Enhancement of transdermal drug delivery by ionophoresis and phorphoresis. *M. Pharm Thesis*, New Delhi. Jamia Hamdard (Supervisor: RK Khar).

8.3.4 Bhatia S (1994) Enhancement of transdermal drug delivery of lignocaine hydrochloride by ionophoresis and ibuprofen by prodrug approach. *M Pharm Thesis*, New Delhi, Jamia Hamdard (Supervisor: RK Khar).

8.3.5 Rafi K (1994) Enhancement of transdermal drug delivery of cyclopiroxalamine and diphtheria toxoid by ionotophoresis. *M Pharm Thesis*, New Delhi, Jamia Hamdard (Supervisor: RK Khar).

8.3.6 Sultana Y (1995) Development of an antiaging formulation and its evaluation using mice model. *M Pharm Thesis*, New Delhi, Jamia Hamdard (Supervisor: RK Khar).

8.4 RESEARCH PAPERS (PUBLISHED/PRESENTED)

8.4.1 Srivastava SC, Khan MSY and Vohora SB (1971) Pharmacological and hemostatic studies on *Sphaeranthus indicus* Linn. *Indian J Physiol Pharmac* **15**, 27.

8.4.2 Zafarullah M, Bano H and Vohora SB (1980) *Juzam* (Leprosy) and its treatment in Unani medicine. *Amer J Chinese Med, USA*, **81(4)**, 370.

8.4.3 Vohora SB (1983) Studies on Unani drug *Biskhapra (Trianthema portulacastrum* Linn), *Planta Medica*, Germany **47(2)**, 106.

8.4.4 Vohora SB 91984) *Ayurvedic Research Seminar on Skin Diseases*, Abstract, p. 45, Jamnagar, Gujarat Ayurved University.

8.4.5 Vohora SB (1985) What is purification of Blood? *Hamdard Medicus*, Pakistan, **28(1)**, 72.

8.4.6 Vohora SB (1986) Elementology of leprosy, *Indian J Lepr.* **58(3)**, 451.

8.4.7 Vohora SB and Wani H (1986) A review of antiinflammatory plants. *Herba Hungarica*, Hungary, **26(1)**, 73.

8.4.8 Athar M, Elmets CA, Mukhtar M et al (1989) A novel mechanism for the generation of superoxide anion in porphyrin-mediated cutaneous photosensitization. Activation of xanthine oxidase pathway, *J Clin Invest* USA, **83**, 1137.

8.4.9 Mukhtar H, Merk H and Athar M (1989) Skin chemical carcinogenesis, *Clin Dermatol*, USA, **7**, 1.

8.4.10 Athar M, Llyod JR, Bickers DR et al (1989) Malignant conversion of radiation and chemically induced mouse skin benign tumours by free radical generating compounds. *Carcinogenesis*, USA, **10**, 1841.

8.4.11 Athar M, Mukhtar H, Bickers DR et al (1989) Evidence for the metabolism of tumour promotor organic hydroperoxides into free radicals by human skin keratocytes. An ESR spin tapping study. *Carcinogenesis*, USA, **10**, 1499.

8.4.12 Nontasut C, Athar M, Zaim MJ et al (1989) Evidence for the involvement of superoxide anions in 8-methoxy psoralen mediated cutaneous photosensitivity *in vivo*. *J. Invest Dermatol*, USA **92**, 492.

8.4.13 Mukhtar H, Athar H, Lloyd JR et al (1989) All-trans retinoic acid exerts a novel anticarcinogenic effect by inhibiting malignant conversion of skin papillomas. *J Invest Dermatol*, USA, **92**, 47.

8.4.14 Mukhtar H, Athar M, Agarwal R et al (1990) Chloroaluminum aptholocyanine tetrasulfonate (AIPCTS)-mediated photodynamic therapy in cutaneous tumours. *Photochem Photobiol.*, USA, **51** (Suppl.) 745.

8.4.15 Agarwal R, Athar M, Urban SA et al 91991) Involvement of singlet oxygen in chloraluminum pathalocyanine tetrasulfonate mediated photoenhancement of lipid peroxidation in rat epidermal microsomes. *Cancer Lett*, USA, **56**, 125.

8.4.16 Athar M. Agarwal R, Wang ZY et al (1991) All-trans retinoic acid protects against free radical generating compounds mediated conversion of chemical and ultra violet B radiation-induced skin papillomas to carcinomas. *Carcinogenesis*, USA, **12**, 2325.

8.4.17 Mukhtar H, Agarwal R, Athar M et al (1991) Photodynamic therapy of murine skin tumours using Photofrin II. *Photodermatol Photoimmunol Photomed*, USA, **8**, 169.

8.4.18 Athar M, Ali S, Siddiqui MY et al (1991) Role of reactive oxygen species in cutaneous chemical carcinogenesis. *Intl. J. Toxicol. Occupat, Environ. Hlth.* **1**, 86.

8.4.19 Naqvi SAH, Khan, MSY and Vohora SB (1991) Antibacterial, antifungal and anthelmintic studies on Indian medicinal plants. *Fitoterapia*, Italy **62(3)**, 221.

8.4.20 Dobrowolski JW, Vohora SB. Sharma K et al (1991) Antibacterial, antifungal, antiamoebic, antiinflammatory and antipyretic studies on Propolis bee products. *J. Ethnopharmacology*, Ireland, **35(1)**, 77.

8.4.21 Agarwal R, Athar M, Lewen RL et al (1992) Photodynamic therapy of chemically and ultraviolet radiation-induced murine skin tumours. Comparison of Photofrin II and chloraluminum phthalocyanine tetrasulfonate. *Photochem Photobiol* **54**, 43.

8.4.22 Elmets CA, Athar M, Zaidi SI et al (1992) Contact sensitivity to dimethyl benz(a)anthracene is influenced by the genes within the major histocompatibility complex and receptor locus. *Clin. Res.*, USA, **40A**, 309.

8.4.23 Mirando WS, Athar M, Mukhtar H et al (1992) UV radiations and photosensitizers plus light promote monocyte antimicrobial activities. *Clin Res.* **40A**, 541.

8.4.24 Vohora SB (1994) Skin diseases: two Unani Concepts. *Invited Lecture, XIII Orientation Programme for Drug Inspectors/Drug Analysts in ISM*, Ghaziabad, Pharmacopoeial Laboratory for Indian Medicine.

8.4.25 Giri U, Sharma SD, Abdulla M et al (1995) Evidence that *in situ* generated reactive oxygen species act as potent stage I tumour promotor in mouse skin. *Biochem Biophys Res Commun.* **209**, 698.

8.4.26 Anderson C, Herr A, Robbins R et al (1995) Metabolic requirements for induction of contact hypersensitivity to immunotoxic polyaromatic hydrocarbons. *J. Immunol* **155**, 3530.

8.4.27 Giri U, Iqbal M and Athar M (1996) Porphyrin-mediated photosensitization has a weak tumor promoting effect in mouse skin: Possible role of *in situ* generated reactive oxygen species. *Carcinogenesis* **17**, 2023.

Index